PSYCHOLOGY OF EMOTIONS, MOTIVATIONS AND ACTIONS

POSITIVE HUMAN FUNCTIONING FROM A MULTIDIMENSIONAL PERSPECTIVE

VOLUME 2

PROMOTING HEALTHY LIFESTYLES

Psychology of Emotions, Motivations and Actions

Additional books in this series can be found on Nova's website under the Series tab.

Additional e-books in this series can be found on Nova's website under the e-book tab.

PSYCHOLOGY OF EMOTIONS, MOTIVATIONS AND ACTIONS

POSITIVE HUMAN FUNCTIONING FROM A MULTIDIMENSIONAL PERSPECTIVE

VOLUME 2

PROMOTING HEALTHY LIFESTYLES

A. RUI GOMES
RUI RESENDE
AND
ALBERTO ALBUQUERQUE
EDITORS

nova publishers
New York

For permission to use material from this book please contact us:
Telephone 631-231-7269; Fax 631-231-8175
Web Site: http://www.novapublishers.com

Library of Congress Cataloging-in-Publication Data

ISBN: 978-1-62948-973-5

Published by Nova Science Publishers, Inc. † New York

This book is dedicated to...

...all my family, especially my parents who were persistent in giving me the best life and educational opportunities, and to my wife Ana and daughters Joana and Tiago who give me the best opportunities to be a happy person every day. And I would like to recognize the six years of working together with our research group, "Adaptation, Performance and Human Development", because the insights and constant encouragement of all the members were critical for the success of this book.

A. Rui Gomes

... to Inês and Artur for the meaning they bring to our existence (mine and of Ana, my wife) and the hope they carry to the future.

Rui Resende

... to my parents who, if they were alive, would love to know that this book was finished. This book happened because of them; I owe almost everything to them.

To my wife, Suzana, who has always been the great supporter of my personal and professional life.

To my children (Marta, Tiago, Diana, and João) and grandchildren (Zé, Clara, and Francisco), who are the most important people in my life. The success of this book is also their own success.

I also thank my companions on this journey, Rui Gomes and Rui Resende.

Alberto Albuquerque

CONTENTS

EDITORS' NOTE

THE BOOK

"Positive human functioning from a multidimensional perspective" tries to understand factors involved in the human adaptation to stressful situations, the human adoption of healthy life styles, and the human training for high performance. Considering these main goals, the book is edited in three volumes related to human adaptation, human development, and human training.

For all volumes, the opening chapter is written by Mihaly Csikszentmihalyi. This chapter addresses the fascinating topic titled "Towards a fully functioning humanity", serving as an introduction to how positive psychology can contribute to the flourishing of humanity in the future.

VOLUME 1
POSITIVE HUMAN FUNCTIONING FROM A MULTIDIMENSIONAL PERSPECTIVE: PROMOTING STRESS ADAPTATION

The main goal of this volume is to analyze human adaptation to life situations. Using examples of work and sport contexts, topics related to stress, emotions, and burnout, both from a theoretical and an empirical point of view, are discussed. How to promote positive adaptation to adaptational contexts is addressed by authors Cary Cooper, Michael P. Leiter, Ronald J. Burke, Marc Jones, Thomas Raedeke, Peter Crocker, and many others.

VOLUME 2
POSITIVE HUMAN FUNCTIONING FROM A MULTIDIMENSIONAL PERSPECTIVE: PROMOTING HEALTHY LIFE STYLES

The main goal of this volume is to analyze human development through the life cycle. Using examples of life skills and exercise practice, topics related to how to organize life skills programs for children, youth, and adults and how to assume healthy life styles by doing regular exercise are discussed. How to promote positive development across the life cycle is addressed by authors Martin I. Jones, Daniel Gould, Tanya Forneris, James E. Maddux, Kimberley L. Gammage, Ali A. Weinstein, and many others.

VOLUME 3
POSITIVE HUMAN FUNCTIONING FROM A MULTIDIMENSIONAL PERSPECTIVE: PROMOTING HIGH PERFORMANCE

The main goal of this volume is to analyze human training to achievement contexts. Using examples of developmental and high performance contexts, topics related to talent development, athletes and teams' training for high performance situations, and leaders' training to maximum professional efficacy (including mainly the cases of sports coaches) are discussed. How to coach individuals, teams, and leaders to high performance is addressed by authors Jean Côté, Eduardo Salas, Robert S. Weinberg, Wade Gilbert, Gordon Bloom, Harold Riemer, and many others.

This is the journey through the complexity of human functioning being assumed in this book; it is a broad and deep perspective of the factors involved in human adaptation, human development, and human training. In sum, this book addresses the fundamental challenge referred to by Kennon M. Sheldon in the Preface of this book, namely, how to make things go right in our lives.

PREFACE

It is with great pleasure that I write this preface, in part because it takes me back to some "golden days" of my professional youth. In 1999 I was fortunate enough to be invited to the Akumal conference, which was held on the Yucatan peninsula, in Mexico. This was the conference which formally hatched the positive psychology movement. It was an exciting time, as eminent researchers (such as Martin Seligman, Mihaly Csikszentmihalyi, and Alice Isen) and "promising young scholars" (such as me, Barbara Fredrickson, and Sonja Lyubomirsky) debated how to proceed. We considered topics such as whether "positive psychology" was the right name for the movement; whether positive psychology was just about people, or whether it should also about relationships, organizations, and institutions; whether positive psychology should have a manifesto, and if so, what should be in it; whether positive psychology was just humanism in a different guise; whether our group itself was too elitist, as we enjoyed our luxury accommodations in a tropical paradise; and much more. Although in subsequent years there were two further conferences held at Akumal, none matched the first for intensity and novelty.

Today, 15 years later, I am very pleased that the positive psychology movement has continued to expand and develop. The robustness of the movement is a testament to people's desire for, and even hunger for, positive psychological perspectives. Twentieth century psychology focused overmuch on human problems, difficulties, errors, and pathologies. It produced manuals for fixing what can go wrong in life, which of course is a depressingly long list. But what about a 21st century "owner's manual" for making things go right in life, for doing what we want? The owner's manuals of our cars do not mainly tell us how to fix problems; instead, they tell us how to operate the car, to do what we want (e.g., how to use the variable-intermittent windshield wiper function, how to check and change the oil). Typically, there is a much shorter problem-solving section at the end of such manuals.

Similarly, the owner's manual for operating human beings could potentially be much longer, or at least more important, than the manual for fixing human beings. This might occur in part because when humans function well, many so-called "problems" evaporate or fix themselves of their own accord. Human misery is in part a function of maladaptive forms of interpreting, construing, and coping with ongoing experience. One enduring premise of positive psychology is that the right sort of "mental tune-up" can sometimes get people to simply replace their maladaptive ways of experiencing, with much more adaptive and proactive ways of experiencing. As one example, a fairly short training in mindfulness meditation can turn a person's experience from feelings of stress, anxiety, and dread of being overwhelmed and unmasked, to a recognition that these feelings are possibilities only -- possibilities that one now has the tools to avoid or sidestep. This new and more adaptive way of encountering stress, rather quickly learned, can sometimes quickly transform an anxious, flustered approach to a much more confident approach to the tasks at hand. Maybe it is better to let problems resolve naturally, rather than try to apply a band-aid to each problem – better to find a single global solution, rather than a host of patches and stop-gaps.

In short, positive psychology is dedicated to balancing the psychological research equation by focusing on human strengths, virtues, health, and happiness in addition to human weaknesses, failings, sicknesses, and unhappiness. And it is working: a recent search found more than 3500 "hits" in PsychInfo for the topic "positive psychology," a number which does not even include the thousands of articles and chapters that address positive psychology themes and topics (happiness, strengths, virtues, skills, capacities) without explicitly referencing the term positive psychology. In addition, dozens of books have been published on positive psychology, including my own "Optimal Human Being: An integrated multilevel perspective" (Sheldon, 2004), "Self-determination theory in the clinic: Motivating mental and physical health" (Sheldon, Williams, & Joiner, 2001) and "Designing positive psychology: Taking stock and moving forward" (Sheldon, Kashdan, & Steger, 2011).

This brings me to the special pleasure of introducing this book with three volumes. As a researcher I have long been interested in what promotes optimal functioning and the highest degree of happiness in individuals. I have mostly taken a personality perspective on this question, focusing on peoples' goals, values, identities, traits, motives, psychological needs, narratives, and more. Typical research studies of mine attempt to predict change in some positive individual outcome (i.e., well-being, happiness, resilience, need-satisfaction) from prior changes in some positive personality characteristic (i.e., goal-attainment, value change, identity development) or from some other positive experience (i.e., a mindfulness intervention, a goal planning procedure, a positive activity induction). Interested readers might see my book "Optimal human being: A integrated multi-level perspective" (Sheldon, 2004) for a summary of conclusions regarding what personality, social, and cultural characteristics are most conducive to promoting human health and wellness.

The authors in the current book, *Positive human functioning from a multidimensional perspective*, have addressed the very same types of question, while taking a somewhat different route. The book has three volumes, each of which addresses optimal human functioning in a particular way. In the first section the book addresses positive human adaptation, in an abstract sense. This includes personality processes but also a variety of other processes, from biological to social. However, there is a twist: the authors focus on adaptation primarily in work and sport contexts, two very important achievement settings for human beings. Thus, there is very tangible, applied angle taken throughout the book, meaning that the book is not just a set of airy abstractions. The second volume of the book addresses positive development, as derived from the positive processes discussed in the first section. Especially at work and in sport, how can people be helped to develop a healthy style of life, one which maximizes their achievement potential and also maximizes their physical and psychological health? The third volume is the most concrete of all, addressing specific training techniques to human performance: how to teach and train individuals, teams, and leaders to best adapt to the present, and best develop in the future. Thus the book leads the reader through the entire process of understanding the nature of positive adaptation, understanding the ways in which positive development occurs given this nature, and understanding the specific ways that this information may be applied for the benefit of real individuals. I commend the editors for settling on this framework, and expect that the book will be popular with a wide spectrum of audiences ranging from theorists to researchers to clinicians to practitioners to teachers, coaches, and even parents. In fact, I can't wait to get my own copy!

Kennon M. Sheldon
Department of Psychology
University of Missouri, Columbia, USA

References

Sheldon, K. M. (2004). *Optimal human being: An integrated multi-level perspective.* New Jersey: Erlbaum.

Sheldon, K. M., Kashdan, T., & Steger, M. (Eds) (2011). *Designing the future of positive psychology: Taking stock and moving forward.* Oxford University Press.

Sheldon, K. M., Williams, G., & Joiner, T. (2003). *Self-Determination Theory in the Clinic: Motivating physical and mental health.* Yale University Press.

Opening Chapter

In: Positive Human Functioning ... Volume 2 ISBN: 978-1-62948-973-5
Editors: A. R. Gomes, R. Resende and A. Albuquerque © 2014 Nova Science Publishers, Inc.

Chapter 1

TOWARDS A FULLY FUNCTIONING HUMANITY

Mihaly Csikszentmihalyi
School of Behavioral and Organizational Sciences, Claremont Graduate University, California, US

ABSTRACT

The chapter reviews briefly the emergence of Positive Psychology in the context of the evolution of psychology as a science, and it suggests how it might contribute to the flourishing of humanity in the future. Focusing on the recently evolved human capacities for self-reflective consciousness and agency, we are now in the position of playing a crucial role in the survival and further evolution of the human species. Whatever decisions we shall collectively take should be informed by a scientific knowledge of the human capacity for creative, constructive – as well as destructive – action, and of the ways these positive capacities can best be applied to shaping a desirable future.

ON THE DEFINITION OF A FUNCTIONING HUMAN

The study of human beings conducted by human beings has adopted the conceptual models and the methods that have served the physical and biological sciences so well in the last few centuries. The followers of the sociology of Auguste Comte or the psychology of B.F. Skinner considered people as organisms that followed behavior patterns established by external stimuli. Men and women had little or no choice over their destiny. The discoveries of Darwin and later those of genetics added even more weight to a reductionist determinism in the study of humanity. The quip attributed to an eminent life scientist: "Molecules are real. All the rest is sociology" is symptomatic of how too many "hard" scientists dismiss explanations of what men and women do that are not based on the most elementary units of organic matter.

Yet, just as biology cannot be reduced to chemistry without losing sight of what makes life different from inorganic processes, so we cannot reduce human life to the simplest organic processes without losing sight of the unique properties of human existence. These properties must include the development of the frontal and pre-frontal cortices – a result of slow biological evolution – which in turn made possible the emergence of *consciousness*, which is an attribute not yet found outside our species. In many ways it is more accurate to say about humans that: "Consciousness is real. All the rest is biology".

Of course, trying to define consciousness is a controversial matter – not surprisingly, since it is such a late gift of evolution. In this context I want to focus on a minimalist definition; by consciousness I mean the information in the mind that is available to our attention. So it includes early genetic instructions like hunger, fear, and sexual attraction. But it also includes our earliest individual memories, the instructions of our parents and our tribe. And it includes learned responses to beauty, to values like generosity or courage. And above all else, consciousness includes the ability to choose from the information it contains a course of action that would not be always predictable even if we had perfect knowledge of the individual's genetic instructions or previous experience (Csikszentmihalyi, 1993).

For a long time, however, the social sciences, and psychology in particular, have tried to ignore the inconvenience that consciousness introduced into the familiar mechanistic conception of the universe that Galileo, Newton, and Leibnitz had so elegantly developed to account for the movements of planets and of molecules. And of course the social sciences have discovered many interesting and important things about the human species. For instance, that most of the time we act as if we were simple robots programmed for self-aggrandizement, for getting the most pleasure available, for using violence and deceit to reach predictable, selfish goals.

Impressed by its own sagacity, the social sciences have then drawn the conclusion that people, like billiard balls, were simply pushed one way or another by outside forces. Of course the forces acting on humans were much more varied and conflicting than those typically propelling billiard balls; but the general idea was by and large the same. So to make matters simple, many of our colleagues concluded that consciousness and its derivatives were merely epiphenomena they could safely dismiss. Ignoring the last few tens of thousands of years of evolution, they found the keys to human action in the behavior of rats and monkeys, while forgetting the wise words attributed to Albert Einstein; "Make things as simple as possible, but not simpler."

The first psychological laboratory, founded by Wilhelm Wundt in Leipzig about a hundred years ago, tried to make the measurement of human behavior as simple as possible concentrating on neurological and muscular response-times; his followers on both sides of the Atlantic followed in his footsteps – arguably reducing the study humankind to something that is too simple to reveal the range of human possibilities.

Of course, there have been many eminent psychologists, ranging from Carl Jung to Abraham Maslow and Karl Rogers, who felt that in pursuing simple rigor psychology had made a bad bargain. Nevertheless, almost all the young people entering graduate programs in psychology were taught that the future of the discipline required that they become more and more reductionist, until they reached the blessed state of technicians dressed in white gowns, who work surrounded by microscopes, computers, and the latest paraphernalia of high technology.

Yet as time passed it became increasingly obvious that there were many questions the 20th century paradigm of psychology had a hard time resolving. For instance Roy Baumeister, a noted social psychologist, asked himself how it was possible for so many new ideas, lifestyles, technologies to appear in human history if everything we did was a product of the past. Clearly the intervention of human consciousness must be a game changer, creating novelties that arose from imagination as well as from the past. He and Marty Seligman (a staunch behaviorist in his youth) developed the notion of *prospection* to account for that part of human action that was determined not only by the past, but also by future goals anticipated in the mind (Seligman, Railton, Baumeister, & Sripada, 2013). Behaviors such as generosity, filial piety, patriotism, altruism might be built on inheritance and learning, but become actual influences on conduct when they are named, defined, and taught.

Baumeister (2008) went so far as resuscitating the long discredited concept of *free will*, arguing that the belief in conscious choice was by itself a recently evolved causal factor in human action. If you believed you had a choice, this belief allowed you to choose between the various options – overriding, if necessary, both the genetic and the social instructions programmed in consciousness.

In fact, ignoring this new development in the functioning of the brain – the ability to make choices among alternatives – leads to untenable results. If people have no other options than to simply act out the instructions contained in their genes or their environment, it would make no sense to hold them responsible for their actions. Instead of relatively autonomous agents, people would be seen as complex robots. Then a well-functioning human being would be one that went through life satisfying his biologically programmed needs as much as possible, while interfering as little as possible with the needs of other human beings. In many ways this would not be such a bad definition, yet it seems to fall far short of the image of man that we are used to. Not to mention that the logic of this simple definition allows individuals who are convinced of their genetic superiority to dominate and exploit the rest of the population in order to satisfy their own requirements for wellbeing. Recent history has shown what can happen when the megalomania of a Hitler or a Stalin becomes translated into public policy.

The view of what a well-functioning person is like is quite different in the emerging perspective of positive psychology. Human beings are seen as a work in progress; tied by strong bonds to the past, but acquiring new powers due to both biological and to cultural evolution. Of course there is no guarantee that this process will have a positive outcome. It will depend in large part on our own decisions whether the future will be flourishing or dismal. But the first step towards a better future is to realize that we can choose, and that it is our choices that will make the difference. So a fully functioning human being, according to this perspective, is a person who accepts his or her unique position in history, with all the bio-social facticity attached, and accepts the responsibility to work for a future in synchrony with the arc of evolutionary movement towards higher levels of complexity. In other words, a fully functioning human being accepts responsibility for piloting spaceship earth.

My Personal Journey to Positive Psychology

The considerations described in the previous sections, important as they are, were not the main reasons that I became dissatisfied with the psychology of the past century. The reasons were much less rational and more experiential. As a child during World War II, I saw some people act with honesty and dignity, others with craven selfishness. I knew that my father, who was the Hungarian consul in the Italian city of Fiume (now Rijeka, in Croatia), was issuing visas and passports to fugitives trying to escape from the Fascist authorities, even though we knew that his superiors in the State Department might fire or even have him imprisoned for flaunting the official policy. He did not ask for payment for this service, in fact he sometime had to lend his own money to people who had not the means to make an escape. By the time I was ten years old, the entire social, cultural, economic, and political system collapsed; relatives (including my older brother Károly) were killed; people lost their jobs, property – and all too often, their reason for living. It seemed to me that some of the adults I knew made choices that kept them sane, efficient, and helpful to others – while others made choices that left them bitter and useless to themselves and everyone else.

In the midst of all the shooting, the fires, the fear and the hunger I made an unexpected discovery. An older cousin taught me how to play chess. After learning the basic moves, I found that the game had such a power over my mind that I hardly noticed a building collapse across the street, or a burst of machine-gun bullets miss the window by inches. I learned something that 30 years later I found out philosophers from Heraclitus to Plato and down to Nietzsche and Sartre had remarked on for many centuries: play provides an alternative reality where we can feel in harmony with the world, and feel more free than at any time in "real" life.

Later on, I had the same experience while mountain climbing, or playing soccer and basketball. All these "games" were able to limit reality to a playing field and a set of rules for action, providing a small world sheltered from the larger world; a small world where one could act with clear purpose and full engagement. A few years later I discovered that the same experience of full concentration could be had from activities where you made up your own purpose, determined your own goals: for instance painting, writing short stories, or even when reading a good novel that forced you to imagine how it would be to be the character in the story, in a place and a time different from the one your body happened to be in.

By the time I was 20 years old, I had decided to become a psychologist, to understand better why some people could live relatively happy lives, while others were just marking time in misery. This was not easy to do in post-war Europe, especially for someone like me who had dropped out of high school at age 14 in order to work and survive. After a long wait for a visa, I entered the USA at age 22, with $1,25 in my pocket, found a nighttime job as a cashier in a large Chicago hotel, while during the day I worked on a BA in psychology at the University of Illinois, where I was admitted after taking an equivalency exam.

But the psychology being taught in the mid-50s was not what I had expected after having read the works of Carl Jung in Europe. It was a discipline that prided itself on its objectivity, seeing human behavior as no different from the behavior of the great apes, or even rats. It indulged in what the social philosopher Hannah Arendt has called the "debunking perspective" of the social sciences emerging out of the older natural sciences, eager to demonstrate their own scientific rigor. Many times over the next ten years I was tempted to leave the study of psychology, and do something less fanciful: like become a forest ranger, or a fiction writer (I had been able to place two short autobiographical stories that I wrote for an English language class in the elite literary magazine *The New Yorker*). For better or for worse, with the help of some wise and understanding teachers at the University of Chicago where I transferred, I went on to finish my doctorate – after which I was hired to teach sociology and anthropology (two subjects that interested me, but had taken just one course in each during my academic career) at a small but vibrant liberal arts college. I taught there for five years, then was invited back to the faculty of the prestigious University of Chicago, where I slowly developed the concept of *flow* and the systems model of creativity, in an effort to move psychology in a direction that was closer to what I thought it should be.

The Public Story of the First Ten Years of Positive Psychology

In the winter of 1998, my wife and I booked a week's vacation at a resort on the Kona Coast of Hawaii. By a rare coincidence, the second day of our stay Martin Seligman and I almost literally ran into each other at a nearby beach. We had met before at psychology meetings, but never had a chance to really talk. Now it turned out that he and his family were staying at the same resort we were. So for the next few days, from breakfast to after dinner, we exchanged ideas about our profession. This was the year before Marty became President of the APA, and he was aware that a once-in-a-lifetime opportunity to leave a legacy was about to open for him.

Even though our training and life experiences were quite different, we soon felt that our views of where psychology should be moving were very similar. We both felt that the reductionist model of man that psychologists, in their desire to appear hard-nosed scientists, had been following for the past few generations, was missing the point. After they discovered behind the veil of Victorian pieties that human beings were obeying instincts inherited from ancestors indistinguishable from apes, psychologists were left with the conclusion that human behavior was *nothing but* animal behavior. The accomplishments that we are so proud of, like the use of language that resulted in the works of Homer, Dante, Shakespeare, or Goethe, are simple side-effects of an evolutionary pattern based on complex thought processes that were selected because they gave our species an advantage in the struggle for survival. Similarly love, gratitude, courage, spirituality, are not things we cherish for their own sake, but because they help us endure, survive, and reproduce.

Neither Marty nor I were comfortable with this. Somewhere the baby had been thrown out with the bathwater. The development of the pre-frontal cortex in humans had been a game-changer; people have developed internal representations of goals they hope for, things they desire and love – and these have become real and important in determining their behavior. It was time, we felt, for psychologists to take seriously the whole spectrum of human functioning, not just the part of it we share with our simian ancestry.

Of course, by then many people outside of psychology and some within it had come to the same conclusion. The teachings of Maslow and Rogers, which spawned Humanistic Psychology, are eloquent examples. However, we felt that the critique of scientism usually falls into the opposite extreme, ignoring the insights of science while rejecting its misapplied reductionism. So where did that leave us? We decided to try formulating our views in a way that our colleagues in the profession would feel compelling. But the effects of whatever we wrote would take years to bring fruit, and by then Marty's presidency would long be over. How could we implement what we thought was an important enrichment of the science of psychology within a shorter span of time?

It was at this point that my PhD thesis and subsequent publications on creativity began to suggest some choices – even though, at the time, I was not consciously aware of it (Csikszentmihalyi, 1996; Getzels & Csikszentmihalyi, 1976). What I knew – based on

Thomas Kuhn's work with the rise of new paradigms in science, and Pierre Bourdieu's analysis of cultural change – was that it is easier to influence the future course of a science by appealing to the curiosity and energy of younger scientists than by trying to influence the already established practitioners, who had much to lose and little to gain from a new perspective that could replace the one in which they had prospered. So instead of appealing to our peers, we decided to invite a small group of young psychologists for a week of meetings, to discuss what these ideas might contribute to the future of psychology.

A few key decisions we made at this point turned out to be inspired. Marty, because of his recent campaigning for the APA Presidency, knew most of the leading psychologists in the country. We decided to write to 50 of these individuals, asking them to nominate a former student less than 30 years of age, who might be sympathetic to our ideas, *and who had a chance to become chairpersons of their psychology departments before they reached the age of* 50. We would then write to the nominated individuals, ask them for their c.v.'s, and invite about twenty to spend a week in a sleepy fishing village Marty knew in Quintana Roo – on the "Mayan Riviera" of Mexico.

This way, we thought, we might kick-start the formation of a *field*. As to the *domain*, -- or the specific content and rules that distinguish one discipline from others -- we thought that there were enough books and articles at the margins of the psychological literature to get things started; the newly constituted field would then take over with the contribution of their own work. If the domain and field turned out to have credibility, it would then attract *persons* to the new sub-domain, which after long deliberations we came to call *Positive Psychology* (Seligman & Csikszentmihalyi, 2000).

The week we spent in the village of Akumal with the twenty young colleagues went by very rapidly, but left an enduring mark on the profession. Of these participants, several (e.g. Barbara Fredrikson, Jonathan Haidt, Corey Keyes, Sonja Ljiubomirski, Ken Sheldon) have written their own book (or books) on various aspects of positive psychology. Practically all of them are still very actively shaping the emerging sub-domain. And they are not alone: the Third World Congress of positive psychology took place in Los Angeles in 2013, with the attendance of about 1500 psychologists form all over the world. It was an unqualified success both in scientific and humane terms. Earlier world congresses have taken place in the United Kingdom and in Philadelphia; European Congresses were held in Stresa, (Italy); Opatija, near Rijeka, the town I was born in, (Croatia); Copenhagen (Denmark), and in the summer of 2012 in Moscow, Russia.

This astonishing growth was made possible in large part because so many young people felt that psychology needed to expand in new directions. Thus our ideas resonated with the spirit of the times. But they needed the exertions of the emerging sub-field to become actualized. Here Marty played an indispensible role. For instance, he was able to secure the financial support of the Templeton Foundation to establish a series of prizes for young scholars in positive psychology, including a yearly $100,000 first prize, which was (and still is) one of the largest monetary recognition for breakthrough research done in psychology. The symbolic significance of such support sent the message that the new sub-domain was not a fleeting affair, but was taken seriously by the world at large. The Meyerson Foundation then helped funding the VIA *Dictionary of Strengths* (intended as the Positive Psychology counterpart to the DSM IV dictionary of psychopathology), spearheaded by Chris Petersen (2006).

Marty also started the highly successful and influential MA program in positive psychology at the University of Pennsylvania, which has inspired similar programs in Denmark, Italy, South Korea, and elsewhere. In 2006 the first PhD program in Positive Psychology was started at the Claremont Graduate University in California. The *Journal of Positive Psychology* also started publishing a few years ago, and is gaining momentum and reputation.

WHAT POSITIVE PSYCHOLOGY CONTRIBUTES TO THE UNDERSTANDING OF HUMAN BEHAVIOR

At this point in its development, Positive Psychology claims to have three main goals. The first is to understand and learn how to improve the momentary affective states of individuals. The second is to study more permanent traits (or "strengths") that some individuals possess, and learn how those who lack them can acquire them. The third addresses the question of how institutions, from families to nation states, might help develop such strengths.

Peterson and Seligman's classification of strengths and virtues (2004) has become one of the main planks of positive psychology. Based on an extensive review of what "virtues" are universal to mankind, it consists of 24 "strengths" grouped in 6 higher-order virtues. Anyone can measure his or her strengths against established norms, and establish their *signature strengths*.

This attempt to single out some traits and calling them *strengths* has caused many lifted eyebrows in the psychological community. Positive psychology has been accused of introducing value judgments in what should be an objective science. But of course psychology, like medicine or even biology, has never been value-free. It has always tried to avoid disease and considered pathology a condition to be changed. What positive psychology has done is simply develop the other end of the continuum from pathology to flourishing, by identifying various kinds of traits and conditions that lead to good physical and mental health. Psychiatrists and psychologists have been turning the pages of the thick tomes of the *Diagnostic and Statistical Manual*, or DSM, which lists the symptoms and possible cures of all that can go awry in the human mind. What Peterson and Seligman did was to try to develop the opposite, which they subtitled *A Dictionary of the Sanities*.

THE FUTURE OF POSITIVE PSYCHOLOGY

The amount of research, publications, meetings and organizations that have been inspired by positive psychology has indeed been incredibly widespread. A simple linear projection into the future would suggest that this "movement" will have hundreds of thousand members in just a few years, and that its influence will permeate institutions around the world, from schools to families, from businesses to governments. History, however, rarely proceeds in a linear direction. Even the history of science is not quite linear: physicists at the beginning of the 20th century thought that their science had exhausted all the mysteries of matter; then in the first quarter of the century the advent of subatomic physics expanded the horizons of the science in unimaginable directions; and by the end of the century physicists had acquired the mantle of the magi of knowledge. Yet only a few decades later new horizons beacon: microbiology, astrophysics, nanotechnologies – to name just a few domains on the ascendant – promise to answer the mysteries of creation.

So whether positive psychology will keep its momentum going is by no means certain. One thing to remember that the higher and swifter a new idea raises, the faster and farther it can fall. The danger with positive psychology is that if too many people expect quick and easy solutions to their lives, and these don't happen, then they turn against the idea and ruin its reputation. Yet many self-styled "life coaches" believe that positive psychology provides a panacea they can promote to clients who are unhappy with their lives. It is important to remember that positive psychology is not a miracle cure. It is simply a perspective that can help scientists advance knowledge in ways that in the fullness of time will allow individuals to improve the quality of their lives. It will not be an easy journey, or a quick one. But it is absolutely necessary that we start on it.

As for what direction Positive Psychology is likely to go in the foreseeable future I must confess ignorance. The problem is that no future course of events is really "foreseeable", especially when it depends on human action. The variables are too many, and too complexly interrelated. I think speculating about what will happen in the future is a worthless exercise.

I do, however, have very strong opinions about what Positive Psychology *should* be trying to accomplish. In fact, my ambitions in that respect are rather extravagant. It seems to me that three main tasks will determine whether humankind will prosper in the future, or cease to exist. I don't know if we will have the vision, and the resolution, to take on these tasks and bring them to a positive resolution. But we have come to a point in the evolution of the species where we can, and we must, take control of our own lives. If we do not, or if we make the wrong choices, we will have only ourselves to blame for our demise.

The first task is to decide *Who We Want To Be*. Each human group that has survived in the past had an idea of what a person should be like, and tried – never with complete success – to educate, train, inspire and force people to come close to that ideal. Cultures changed rather slowly in the past, adjusting their notion of desirable personhood over generations as technologies, political and economic realities changed. The changes that cultures have undergone in the past two generations are more rapid and more radical than they had ever been. On the other hand, the image of what constitutes a good person has not caught up with the new realities. Yet human genetics and biotechnology have now reached the point that we can imagine ordering "designer babies" from illustrated catalogs, with genes tweaked to facilitate learning, or domineering, or nurturing – as well, of course, as hair and eye color. What choices will we make? And who will make them? In a few years, these questions will have to be faced. And Positive Psychology should be in a position to help inform the public discourse on these issues, pointing out the long-term as well as the short-term results of various actions to the self and to the community.

The second task we will have to decide is, *Where do We Want To Live*? On a planet that increasingly resembles a Garden of Eden, or a planet that has become an orbiting garbage can? Which of these outcomes will come true, depends exclusively on us. And again, Positive Psychology should help the other social sciences involved in policies of sustainability and conservation, to show people how their lifestyle habits, and the policies of their elected officials, can create a better world for our grandchildren to live in.

Finally, the last question is, *What Shall We Do*? The cultural changes of the past century have affected every aspect of our lives: What kind of families our children are born into, what education they receive, what opportunities to express themselves they have, what jobs are open for them… and so on and on, until the ever prolonged period of late life, where people feel increasingly useless and abandoned…

In many parts of the world, the normal development of teenagers, and even children, is interrupted and twisted forever by narcotics dealers, diamond smugglers, or sweatshops. In Africa alone, the number of children who are given weapons and taught to kill is estimated at a minimum of 100,000. In the richer and more stable countries of the world, millions of young people, deprived of a context of development and with nothing to do, become prey of illusory chemical solutions. Similarly, untold millions of adults are left without a job, without a role in society. Those fortunate enough to find employment often work at jobs that were not designed to improve the life of workers, but to generate the maximum profit to wealthy investors.

Positive psychology will deserve its place among the great achievements of mankind to the extent that it takes seriously its responsibility to contribute the accumulating knowledge it produces to the solution of these three challenges facing us: To decide who we will be, where will we live, and what will we do.

REFERENCES

Baumeister, R. (2008). *Are we free? Psychology and free will*. New York: Oxford University Press.

Csikszentmihalyi, M. (1993). *The evolving self: A psychology for the third millennium*. New York: Harper/Collins.

Csikszentmihalyi, M. (1996). *Creativity: Flow and the psychology of discovery and invention*. New York: Harper/Collins.

Getzels, J. W. & Csikszentmihalyi, M. (1976). *The creative vision*. New York: Wiley.

Peterson, C. (2006). *A primer in positive psychology*. New York: Oxford University Press.

Peterson, C. & Seligman E. M. (2004) *Character strengths and virtues: A handbook of classification*. New York: Oxford University Press.

Seligman, M. E. & Csikszentmihalyi, M. (2000). Positive psychology: An introduction. *American Psychologist, 55*, 1, 5-14.

Seligman, M. E., Railton, P., Baumeister, R. & Sripada, C. (2013). Navigating into the future or driven by the past. *Perspectives on Psychological Science, 8*(2), 119-141.

LIFE SKILLS

In: Positive Human Functioning ... Volume 2 ISBN: 978-1-62948-973-5
Editors: A. R. Gomes, R. Resende and A. Albuquerque © 2014 Nova Science Publishers, Inc.

Chapter 2

LIFE SKILLS PROGRAMS: WHAT MAKES THEM WORK?

Martin I. Jones and John K. Parker
School of Sport and Exercise,
University of Gloucestershire, Cheltenham, UK

ABSTRACT

The purpose of this chapter is to provide an overview of what we consider to be some important concepts and debates in the current life skill literature and to discuss possible reasons why life skill programs are effective in facilitating optimal human functioning. Specially designed programs that aim to develop the skills needed for everyday life, by everybody, that help people thrive (i.e., life skills) are common in the scientific literature, however not all programs are rigorously evaluated and consequently it is not clear how these programs facilitate development. Researchers and program leaders refer to the power of social relationships as a vehicle for positive development. In this instance, the relationships between the program participants (i.e., peer-to-peer interaction), and the relationships between the program leader and participant (i.e., adult-to-peer interaction) provide the basis for skills to be learned. Researchers also consider the environment in which the program exists to be critically important for individuals to learn skills. For example, researchers have listed the facets of effective life skills programs.

Finally, the ecology of human development (e.g., developmental systems theories) provides a final possible explanation for the effectiveness of life skills programs. From a developmental systems perspective, positive outcomes are the results of numerous bi-directional interactions between the individual and her context underpinned by the plasticity (i.e., potential for change) of the developing person. In this chapter, we review some of the evidence in support of existing mechanisms. We also provide possible areas for discussion including the possibility that life skills programs provide the basis of a crystalizing experience, transfer as a threshold concept, and the possibility that multiplicative models of thriving and life skill development may provide an alternative to the traditional additive models. In closing, we believe that life skill programs can facilitate optimal human functioning; however, scholars and practitioners need to clarify the reasons why life skills programs facilitate optimal human functioning.

INTRODUCTION

> Running taught me valuable lessons. In cross-country competition, training counted more than intrinsic ability, and I could compensate for a lack of natural aptitude with diligence. I applied this in everything I did.
>
> (Nelson Mandela, 1995, p. 55)

One of the oldest debates in psychology revolves around how to help people function optimally and reach their potential. Sir Francis Galton (1869) considered the development of genius nearly 150 years ago, and since then several other eminent psychologists have wrestled with the perennial problem of optimal human functioning. Despite the apparent interest in human functioning, the studies of disease and psychological deficits have dominated the psychology literature. Studies of depression, anxiety, emotional disturbances, and cognitive maladies abound (to name but a few). Even though the deficit paradigm has dominated contemporary psychology researchers interested in the positive sides of psychology have investigated human functioning. Researchers such as Martin Seligman, Mihalyi Cziksentmihalyi, Dean Simonton, Howard Gardner, Richard Lerner, and many others have conducted research that has enabled practitioners to optimize human life, to provide conditions for betterment, and to facilitate thriving.

Richard Lerner and colleagues (Lerner et al., 2006) stated that a person may be said to be thriving if she is involved in healthy, positive developmental regulations (the interaction between an individual and her context) and on the path to idealized personhood, marked by making culturally valued contributions to self, others, and institutions (Csikszentmihalyi & Rathunde,1998). If thriving is the result, what is the process? How can we facilitate thriving?

One such method of personal improvement, which has received attention in the sport and exercise psychology literature, comes in the form of a specially designed life skills program. In the opening quote, Nelson Mandela suggested that sport could teach life skills. In Mandela's case, running taught the lesson of diligence, which he applied to other achievement domains. The link between participation in sport and positive development also has a rich history in scholarly research. For example, a paper by C. H. McCloy (1930) in the first volume of Research Quarterly demonstrated one of the first attempts to outline a process of seeking specific character developments through well-planned activities (i.e., through physical education). Even though this paper is 80 years old, many of the points are still relevant today (Weiss & Gill, 2005).

Other political and religious leaders and philosophers have described the benefits of sport on the development of the person. For example, Plato proclaimed that the moral value of sport far outweighed the physical value. Current President of the International Olympic Committee, Jacques Rogge (2004), said, "The world of sport is not separate from the rest of the world. Sport breaks down barriers, promotes self-esteem, and can teach life skills and healthy behavior." Pope John Paul II (2000) said, "The potential of sports makes it a significant vehicle for the overall development of the person and a very useful element in building a more human society." However, sport can also be a force for bad (e.g., Ogilvie & Tutko, 1971). If adults leave young people without appropriate support, sport can teach negative skills, values, and virtues (e.g., cheating, drug use, and increased rates of alcohol abuse). It may be that practitioners need to teach life skills in a systematic style. Consequently, scholars and practitioners need to consider using specially designed life skills programs. Moreover, scholars and practitioners need evidence based life skills programs that improve human functioning. To this end, the purpose of this chapter is to provide an overview of what we consider to be some important concepts and debates in the current life skill literature and to discuss possible reasons why life skill programs are effective in facilitating optimal human functioning.

What Is a Life Skill?

Gould and Carson (2008) stated that the interest in life skills development through sport, especially in children and youth, clearly exists because most youth sports organizations have social-emotional development as a stated goal. Similarly, Gould and Carson noted an increasing interest in life skills research where scholars and practitioners use sport as a vehicle to teach life skills. Nevertheless, there are several inconsistencies and problems that exist, one of which is a clear definition of what constitutes a life skill.

For most people, positive human functioning comprises defining one's sense of self, discovering skills and interests, developing multifaceted competence, and applying the valuable principles learned in one life domain to another. These behaviors, skills, principles, and attitudes are what Danish, Nellen, and Owens (1996) called 'life skills'. The World Health Organization (WHO, 1999) defined life skills as the ability for adaptive and positive behavior that enables individuals to deal effectively with the demands and challenges of everyday life that lead people toward healthy and productive lives. Researchers loosely group life skills into three categories: cognitive skills for analyzing and using information, personal skills for developing personal agency and managing oneself, and inter-personal skills for communicating and interacting effectively with others (UNICEF, 2003).

In addition to policy driven definitions, Jones and Lavallee (2009) defined life skills as ranges of transferable skills needed for everyday life, by everybody, that help people thrive. Jones and Lavallee (2009) highlighted the need for transferability across life domains as a core definitional concept. Transfer comprises individuals developing skills in one life domain and then utilizing the same skills for the purposes of success in different life domains. For example, if an individual can work in a team in the office, but cannot use teamwork skills in other life domains, teamwork is not a life skill for that individual. Conversely, if an individual takes skills learned from sport and uses them in one or more life domain those skills are life skills. If life skills are transferable to other domains, researchers interested in life skills are essentially trying to predict what a person will do in a given situation, based on what they do in another situation. For example, if someone is diligent in sport, can we use that evidence to predict diligence in the workplace? If the answer is yes, we can label diligence as a life skill.

It is possible that life skills are culturally valued and subjective. Lerner et al. (2006) stated that thriving and the path to thriving might be different across cultures, in different nations, or across epochs. Consequently, there will be cultural and individual differences in what people classify as a life skill. To some, washing, cleaning, and ironing are essential life skills, to others, communication and teamwork are more important. In order to augment the debate of what constitutes a life skill, we would like to add something new, adapted from Simonton's (1999) definition of talent. Simonton defined talent as "any innate capacity that enables and individual to display exceptionally high performance in a domain that requires special skills and training" (p. 436). We believe that life skills could be innate (i.e., inherited) but heritability is not a defining feature because some dispositional skills require refinement through training (e.g., deliberate practice) and some life skills will not be inherited. We also believe that life skills allow individuals to demonstrate competence, which could be cognitive, emotional, or behavioral, in a domain (or domains), however the level of performance does not need to be exceptionally high (i.e., elite level of athletic accomplishment). The core concept that applies to life skills is special skills and training. By adapting Simonton's work, we believe that a life skill could enable an individual to display competence in one or more life domains (i.e., they are transferable) that requires special skills and/or training. In this case, brushing one's teeth is a valuable skill, but not a life skill because one does not use teeth brushing to demonstrate competence. Moreover, for most people, brushing ones teeth does not require special skills or training and the skill is not valuable across life domains.

Life Skills in the Context of Human Functioning

> We can, through the application of our science, serve our worlds' citizens; actualize the idea that there is nothing of greater value to society than science devoted to using its scholarship to improve the life chances of all people.
> (Richard Lerner, 2005, p. 57)

Jelicic, Theokas, Phelps, and Lerner (2007) have suggested that the application of rigorously designed interventions can enhance positive human functioning if those interventions align the strengths of individuals and contexts (i.e., positive developmental regulation). As such, practitioners require research that examines the characteristics of individuals and their contexts.

According to UNICEF (2003), life skills education programs are theory and evidence-based, learner-focused, delivered by competent facilitators, and appropriately evaluated to ensure continuous improvement of documented results. To date, several evaluations of life skills programs exist, however, we believe that it is worth noting that there are limited numbers of rigorous, well-designed studies that have tested whether life skills programs work. Although it is not our intention to act as the "methods police" and/or to cast aspersions on fellow researchers, it is important to note that few extant studies demonstrate the highest levels of methodological rigor (e.g., longitudinal studies, randomized control trials, and Meta analyses). Furthermore, they might not include the necessary procedural information to clarify the control and experimental conditions, variations (e.g., intensity, mode of delivery, personnel who deliver it, frequency of delivery, duration of delivery, timing of delivery), or possibility of co-intervention (e.g., coaching and life skills education). As such, readers may view the debate on why life skills programs work as conjecture. Despite this assertion of speculation, several theorists have considered possible mechanisms of life skill development.

In terms of the context, several authors have also described the features of effective interventions. For example, Lerner (2004) described the "Big Three" features of optimal youth development programs. Lerner suggested that youth programs (e.g., life skills programs) are most likely to promote thriving when they involve possibilities for sustained adult-youth relationships, skill-building activities, and opportunities for youth participation in leadership of community-based activities. Catalano, Berglund, Ryan, Lonczak, and Hawkins (1998) found that the majority (about 75%) of effective positive youth development programs focus on Lerner's "Big Three" features of effective programs. Catalano et al. (1998) classified positive development programs as any youth based program that promoted bonding, resilience, competence, self-determination, spirituality, self-efficacy, clear and positive identity, belief in the future, provided recognition for positive behavior and opportunities for prosocial involvement, and prosocial norms. Based on their definition Catalano and colleagues examined the design and outcomes of youth programs in a variety of contexts (e.g., school, family, and community). Catalano and colleagues included published and unpublished programs as long as the authors of the program sampled youth between the ages of 6 and 20 years that were selected because they did not need treatment for a specific mental illness. Catalano et al. excluded delinquency, drug-abuse, and mental-health treatment programs. The interventions had to address at least one youth development construct (e.g., a life skill) in multiple life domains, address multiple youth development constructs in a single life domain, or address multiple youth development constructs in multiple domains. In addition, the authors of the studies or programs needed to demonstrate rigor through appropriate study design and outcome measures, adequate description of the research methodologies, description of the population served, description of the intervention, description of implementation, and effects demonstrated on behavioral outcomes. Based on the aforementioned rigor criteria, cognitive and emotional life skill programs would have been neglected. Even so, Catalano and colleagues provided a comprehensive review of positive development programs.

Catalano et al. (1998) identified 161 programs that met the initial inclusion criteria. Of these programs, 77 had evaluations that Catalano and colleagues tentatively deemed rigorous enough to include in the final analysis. The remaining 84 programs were not included for one of the following reasons: no evaluation existed; the evaluation contained no data beyond a narrative case study; the study sample was an indicated population (symptomatic or in treatment), or adequate evaluation information could not be retrieved.

On closer inspection, Catalano et al. (1998) removed eight more programs from the review because they were sufficiently limited by missing information. Furthermore, the research team removed a further thirty-nine programs that did not have adequate evaluations and five did not have positive effects on behavioral outcomes. The final 25 programs had strong evaluation designs (experimental or quasi-experimental with viable comparison groups), had an acceptable standard of statistical proof, provided adequate methodological detail to allow an independent assessment of the study's soundness, and produced evidence of significant effects on behavioral outcomes. The most effective programs addressed a wide range of positive objectives rather than concentrating on just one area. Similarly, the best programs were rigorously evaluated, made assessments of positive and problem outcomes, had a structured curriculum, lasted for a minimum of nine months, and had high implementation conformity.

The characteristics of effective programs identified by Catalano et al. (1998) are similar to those identified by Roth and Brooks-Gunn (2003). Roth and Brooks-Gunn noted that effective programs transcend an exclusive focus on the prevention of risky behaviors to include attempts to instill behaviors that emphasize youth competencies and abilities (e.g., life skills) through increasing exposure to supportive and empowering environments where activities create opportunities for both skill-building and horizon-broadening experiences. In addition, Roth and Brooks-Gunn (2003) indicated that effective programs offer opportunities for youth to nurture their interests and talents, practice new skills, and gain a sense of personal and group recognition.

Finally, the National Research Council and Institute of Medicine (NRCIM, 2002) outlined eight features of settings that are most likely to foster these developmental assets. According to the NRCIM positive development programs, should be physically and psychologically safe, have appropriate structure, have supportive relationships, provide opportunities to belong, provide positive social norms, support efficacy, and significance, provide opportunities for skills building, and integrate family, school, and community efforts.

In closing, it is evident that for life skills programs to work, program authors need to consider a wide range of program characteristics the researchers in the field of positive youth development have shown to positively influence developmental outcomes.

SOCIAL INTERACTIONS AND THE DEVELOPMENT OF LIFE SKILLS

> The teacher-student relationship is the most important [theme]. Without a certain kind of relationship, nothing else, not integrating personal and social responsibility into physical education, not empowerment, not transfer to the wider world – will work very well. "Show me a good curriculum and a mediocre teacher" as I've often said "and I'll show you a mediocre program."
> (Don Hellison, 2003, p. 97)

It is unlikely that young people develop life skills in a linear system where each skill unfolds in a predictable biologically driven sequence. It is our contention that when young people participate in life skills programs, the skills emerge because of the interactions that occur with that specific context. Developmental psychologist Lev Vygotsky (1962) suggested that development could not be separated from the context in which it occurs. Shabani, Khatib, and Ebadi (2010) noted that Vygotsky, in his genetic law of development, stated that any higher mental function (e.g., a life skill) goes through an external social stage in its development before becoming an internal function. Vygotsky (1978) coined the term zone of proximal development to describe the current or actual level of a learner's development and the next level attainable using tools and adult or peer facilitation. In terms of life skills development, individuals learn best when working alongside other people during collaboration. Furthermore, when individuals collaborate with persons that are more skilled learners learn and internalize new concepts, psychological tools, and skills (i.e., life skills). In essence, a life skills program works because leaders give learners tasks that are too difficult for one person to accomplish alone. In order to complete a given task learners need to collaborate with peers or program leaders. After a successful collaboration, the learner could be better equipped to complete the task individually the next time he or she is exposed to a similar challenge. Through that process, the individual's zone of proximal development, for that particular task, will have been raised. A leader can then promote skill progression by repeating the task at a higher level of difficulty in line with the new zone of proximal development of the learner.

Jones (2012) stated that life skills program leaders scaffold participant's experiences by providing structured practice, by offering motivational support and encouragements, by providing challenge, and steering young people away from potentially frustrating situations. It is worth noting that the leader and participant relationship is bi-directional in nature (i.e., developmental regulation), therefore readers should not confuse scaffolding with a one-way communication process. When scaffolding participants experiences, life skills leaders could consider the quality of the leader-participant interaction and promote bi-directionality rather than purely adult driven direct instruction.

Petitpas, Cornelius, Van Raalte, and Jones (2005) also discussed social relationships in the formation of life skills. Petitpas and colleagues proposed a framework for youth psychosocial development through sport organized into four key areas: context, external assets, internal assets, and evaluation. The context in which youth sport programs exist should be engaging so youth participate because they want to as opposed to because they have to. Program leaders could give young people the opportunity to experiment with new roles and experience the excitement of learning new skills in physically and psychologically safe environments. Finally, program leaders could give young people the opportunity to challenge themselves to maximize a young person's capabilities. External assets include caring adults and a positive group or community. These external assets do not focus on reducing problems but on supporting and promoting success. These people provide opportunities to gain confidence in abilities and to use those abilities in non-sport domains (i.e., facilitate transferability). Internal assets include life skills and values that program leaders teach in a systematic manner that also include strategies for transferability.

Fraser-Thomas, Côté, and Deakin (2005) presented a similar model of sport programming for positive youth development. Their model incorporated talent development research (e.g., Côté, 1999; Côté & Hay, 2002) into a larger framework of positive youth development. Essentially, the model suggests that successful positive youth development programs consider youth's intellectual, physical, psychological, and social stages of development. Programs could be conducted in appropriate settings and they could foster developmental assets. Furthermore, Fraser-Thomas et al. highlighted the importance of policy makers and sports organizations, and suggest key stakeholders ensure accessibility of youth sport programs to all youth, with programs designed to improve youth holistically rather than simply producing better skilled individuals. Finally, Fraser-Thomas and colleagues proposed that it is the responsibility of policy makers and organizations to provide coaches and parents with opportunities to learn and teach internal assets through training, education, and experience so that they can be used as a resource (i.e., external assets). In sum, Fraser-Thomas et al. promote a multi-agent approach in supporting positive youth development through sport.

In both cases (e.g., Petitpas et al., 2005 and Fraser-Thomas et al., 2005) the relationship between program leaders and program participants is a potential explanatory factor in the efficacy of a youth development (e.g., life skills) program. Petitpas, Cornelius, and Van Raalte (2008) stated that development programs are only as effective as the adults that deliver them. Consequently, program leaders who are not able to build trusting relationships with program participants are less likely to create an environment where participants experiment with new roles and experience the excitement of learning new skills in physically and psychologically safe environments. Rhodes (2004) stated that effective programs produce positive outcomes both directly (through close bonds and exposure to programs and instruction) and indirectly (through the staff's establishment of a supportive interpersonal climate characterized by warmth, respect, and friendship). Rhodes also suggested that the relationship between program leader and participant is the essential ingredient in developing an effective life skills program. Rhodes believed that leaders of after school programs, such as a life skills program, are able to engage young people in informal conversations and enjoyable activities that may be limited by the power hierarchy that exists in school settings. Because life skills leaders are typically not the young person's parent or teacher, they are able to provide a safe context for support and guidance and they are able to transmit adult values, advice, and perspectives without the constraints of busy teaching and/or working schedules.

Specific outcomes, such as social and emotional competencies can be developed through attachments between leaders and participants that help participants realign their conceptions of themselves in relation to others. Moreover, leaders can provide participants with opportunities for experimenting with different modes of communication and leaders can help participants to express and control emotions. In doing so, Rhodes (2004) stated that program leaders could help participants better understand, express, and regulate positive and negative emotions and provide a model of effective adult communication, arguably two important life skills.

Despite the possibility that the leader-participant interaction is an essential element in the participant's development of life skills, few studies specifically examine interpersonal relationships as a determinant of positive outcomes (e.g., life skills). That said several authors have discussed how a coach may influence the development of life skills through organized sport.

The Coach Education Approach to Life Skill Development

Proponents of the coach education approach to life skill development base their beliefs on an assertion that teaching coaches how to structure their coaching in a developmentally appropriate manner is the best way to develop life skills in young people. By educating coaches, young people will have positive sport experiences and develop the desirable skills and assets that will help them develop. Thus, it is important to recognize the influence of the coach when examining life skill development.

Conroy and Coatsworth (2006) recommended coach education as an avenue for positive human functioning based on a review of efficacy trials of Coach Effectiveness Training (Barnett, Smoll, & Smith, 1992; Smith, Smoll & Barnett, 1995; Smith, Smoll, & Curtis, 1979; Smoll & Smith, 1984; Smoll, Smith, Barnett, & Everett, 1993) and the Penn State Coaching Training program (Coatsworth & Conroy, 2006; Conroy & Coatsworth, 2004). Conroy and Coatsworth's review revealed that coach education could change coach behavior, particularly increases in reward and reinforcement. Moreover, specific coach education resulted in changes in youths' perceptions of coaches, with Coach Effectiveness Training coaches in particular offering more reward and reinforcement, mistake contingent encouragement, and general technical instruction. Young people who experienced coaching from Coach Effectiveness Training coaches liked their coach more and they believed the coach liked them more. Finally, coach education programs can enhance youth's self-esteem and achievement goals, and reduce youth's anxiety. Conroy and Coatsworth concluded that coach education, with an emphasis on psychosocial education, is an efficacious method for promoting positive development (i.e., positive human functioning).

McCallister, Blinde, and Weiss (2000) also believed that the coach was the most significant individual in terms of life skills development because coaches are in positions of authority and influence and coaches' principles and coaching philosophies will directly influence the experiences of the children and adolescents in their charge. If coaching is effective, McCallister et al. believed that coaches could be instrumental in developing fair play, respect for others, cooperation, decision-making, leadership, and moral development in young people. McCallister et al. interviewed 22 volunteer youth coaches to understand how they developed life skills in their athletes. Results suggested that many coaches assumed that life skills would be an automatic byproduct of participation. If life skills were not a natural byproduct of sport participation, many coaches found it difficult to teach life skills.

Gould, Collins, Lauer, and Chung (2005) extended McCallister and colleagues preliminary investigation by purposefully sampling award winning coaches recognized for their achievements in developing good citizens, productive individuals, and successful athletes. Unlike, McCallister et al., Gould and colleagues' study aim was to understand the strategies coaches use to develop life skills in actual sports programs. Gould et al. described a process of life skills development that was contingent upon a continual process guided by a philosophical base, trust, and strong coach-player relationships. The coaches also implemented specific strategies and follow-up procedures for helping their players develop life skills. Based on the coaches' descriptions of their sporting programs, Gould and colleagues suggested a win at all costs philosophy could be detrimental to the development of life skills whereas a philosophy based on advancing psychosocial development could augment life skill development. These authors stated that a strong coach-athlete relationship, built through communication, empathy, and rapport relationships is integral when developing life skills. Furthermore, using specific strategies, such as treating players with respect and teambuilding, and utilizing resources and environmental considerations, such as parents, peers, and societal norms, allowed the coach to refine life skills in his athletes.

Gould, Chung, Smith, and White (2006) also investigated the role of the coach in developing life skills. Gould et al. surveyed 154 North American high school coaches from seven sports on demographics, coaching objectives, the role of sport in character development, problems in sport today, the role of coaches, and coach influences on athletes. Problems associated with sport today included athletes failing to take personal responsibility, lack of motivation, poor communication skills, problems with parents, and poor grades. Coaches felt they most often took on the role of counselor and athletic trainer, they felt they were prepared to handle these roles, were most successful in fulfilling them, and they felt they were part of their role as a coach. Finally, coaches reported the view that they had considerable influence on the values and behaviors of their athletes and indeed did influence the values and behaviors of their athletes.

Coaches ranked "helping young people develop psychologically and socially" as the most important coaching objective and rated "having a winning team" as least important coaching objective. Coaches reported a belief that sport teaches many life skills. For example, teamwork, the value of hard work, time management, and goal setting are developed through sport participation, however, coaches did not think that sport could refine moral character (e.g., teach fairness, accepting defeat gracefully, or not holding a grudge after competition).

As a direct consequence of the accumulation of literature focused upon the coach's role in developing life skills, Gould and Carson (2008) proposed a five component heuristic model for understanding the process of coaching life skills through sport. The first component of Gould and Carson's (2008) model consists of athletes' existing life skills, personality traits (i.e., internal assets), and exposure to parents, siblings, peers, and socioeconomic status (i.e., external assets). Camiré, Trudel, and Forneris (2012) stated that a coach's knowledge of an athlete's internal and external assets is important because athletes beginning life skills programs are not "blank slates." How an athlete enters a life skills program can greatly influence a coach's ability to develop life skills. For example, that age of the athlete may be an important factor to consider in stage one of the model. Jones, Dunn, Holt, Sullivan, and Bloom (2011a) suggested that differences in positive youth development outcomes between a sample of Canadian sport participants and a sample of American rural afterschool program participants could be attributed to differences in age. It is possible that older participants will have more internal and external resources that may influence the "uptake" of life skills, and therefore coaches should not try a one-size fits all approach when working with different age groups.

The second component of Gould and Carson's (2008) model shows coaches that a developmental coaching philosophy, strong relationship skills, competence, and accessibility are critical factors when developing life skills. In the third component of the model, Gould and Carson, attempt to explain how life skill development occurs and how life skills influence the development of athletes. Gould and Carson suggested that the social environment influences the development of life skills by affecting positive identity changes and formation, membership in a positive peer group, and forming attachments with helpful adults (Eccles, Barber, Stone, & Hunt, 2003). Another explanation for why young people develop life skills in sport is based on the belief that life skills are learned because they are useful in a variety of settings. For example, people learn communication because they need communication across life domains.

The fourth component of the model examines the positive and negative outcomes of sport participation and the fifth component of the model discusses the transferability of life skills to non-support settings. If skills are positive, it is natural to want to transfer skills into other life domains. Allied to this, Gould and Carson suggest coaches facilitate transfer by showing young people a skills value and develop confidence in their ability to use the skill in different life domains. Further, through the facilitation of role exploration, provision of help to adjust to failure, by raising awareness of the skill in question, and providing support and feedback during transfer, a skills utility becomes maximized.

In a subsequent study, Camiré et al. (2012) examined high school coaches' philosophies and strategies used to coach life skills and how to transfer life skills from sport into other life domains. Camiré et al. interviewed 9 coaches and 16 student athletes using Gould and Carson's (2005) model of life skill development to frame the results. Results revealed that coaches understood their student athlete's personal characteristics and adopted coaching philosophies based on the promotion of positive functioning. Results also revealed that coaches used specific strategies to teach life skills and actively educated students on the transfer of skills from sport to other life domains. Camiré et al. stated that coaches adapted their coaching based on an individual's existing skills and career objectives. Coaches also moved beyond technical and tactical coaching toward an athlete-centered approach geared toward using sport as a tool for personal development, and that some coach athlete centered philosophies reflected institutional (e.g., school, clubs, national governing bodies) mandates. In terms of specific strategies for life skills development, Camiré et al. stated that the coaches in their study modeled appropriate behavior, used key words, implemented peer evaluation, used volunteer work, recognized and used teachable moments, and taught students how to transfer skills into different life domains.

Developmental Systems Theories Approach to Life Skills Development

Developmental systems theory is not so much a single theory as a set of theoretical and empirical perspectives on the development and evolution of organisms (Robert, Hall, & Olson, 2003). The developmental systems approach has its roots primarily in developmental and behavioral psychology. Developmental systems theories reject the dualities of development (e.g., nature vs. nurture; organism vs. environment; stability vs. instability). Rather, humans have the potential for change during development because of the integration of a number of developmental systems. The developmental systems theoretical model constitutes a new, non-reductionist, integrative, and multidisciplinary approach to describing, explaining, and optimizing human development (Jelicic et al., 2007).

The basic unit of analysis within the developmental system involves a mutually influential relationship between a developing person and a multilevel and changing ecological context (Jelicic et al., 2007). This is represented as a person ↔ context relation. These bi-directional relations constitute developmental regulation. Adaptive developmental regulations emerge when the interactions between the individual and the context advance the well-being of both components (Lerner, Almerigi, Theokas, & Lerner, 2005).

The potential for change (both individual and contextual), known as plasticity, exists as a consequence of mutually influential relationships between the developing person and his biology, psychological characteristics, family, community, culture, physical and designed ecology, and historical niche (Lerner et al., 2005). The plasticity of the developing human is a key aspect of positive youth development (Lerner et al., 2005). Because change is both possible and expected there are means to improve human life. Everybody can achieve this because plasticity is a strength present in all people (Lerner, 2005). The relative plasticity of humans means that practitioners can target the levels of the development system (e.g., organized activities, family, community, and psychological assets) to help design positive youth development interventions (Hansen, Larson, & Dworkin, 2003). From a developmental systems perspective life skills programs work because they combine with the needs and assets of an individual to provide adaptive developmental regulations.

Moving Forward

Gould and Carson (2008) stated that given the infancy of life skill research there is a need for more and better research. We agree that the field is far from saturated and agree with Gould and Carson's assertions for quantitative and qualitative research, development of better measures, examination of program differences, evaluation research, longitudinal research, experimental research, and the identification of mechanisms and transferability still hold true. In addition to the future research directions proposed by Gould and Carson, we would like to use the following section to propose supplementary arguments that could facilitate debate regarding life skills development. We will address three areas for consideration, namely whether life skills programs serve as a crystalizing experience, whether life skills programs provide grounds for understanding threshold concepts, and whether vertical stacking of life skills provides the basis of thriving (vs. a multiplicative model of life skill attainment).

LIFE SKILLS PROGRAMS AS A CRYSTALIZING EXPERIENCE

> The ideal sport model will not be attained until life skills development occurs within and as a result of the sport experience.
>
> (Miller & Kerr, 2002, p. 150)

Jones (2012) suggested that existing models of life skill development might not reflect how young people acquire life skills and actualize thriving in the real world. The idea that adults can charge young people up with skills that a young person can then discharge in a different life domain is erroneous. An alternative model was derived, based on the work of educational researcher Donald Schön (1987), where young people develop skills through experience and then require additional support to understand that they have developed specific skills (and that these skills are relevant to other life domains). From this perspective, people learn life skills through experience and those experiences are then supplemented with a life skills program that serves a crystalizing experience.

Experiential learning involves learning by doing and then reflecting on the process. Experiential education is based on the belief that active learning is more valuable for the learner because the learner is directly responsible for, and involved in the process. Proponents of this approach believe that learning is a result of direct experience, and includes the premise that people learn best when they have multiple senses actively involved in learning (Crisp, 1998). Individuals learn when placed outside their comfort zones and into a state of dissonance. Learning is then assumed to occur through the changes required to bring the individual back into balance and achieve personal equilibrium (Crisp, 1998).

Schön (1987) presented a theory of experiential learning that emphasized looking to our experiences and connecting with our feelings. Schön's theory of experiential learning and reflective practice has been suggested to stand apart from the other theories of learning because it centers on the construction of domain specific knowledge, through the context of professional practice (i.e., learning via personal experiences). Schön denounced technical rationality as the grounding of knowledge, suggesting it is an inappropriate practice in a dynamic world. Schön compared learning through technical rationality to the charging of a battery. He suggested this positivist epistemology of practice, which aimed to charge people up with information in training so that people can discharge information in practice, is not an accurate representation of how people think and act (Schön, 1987). As such, Schön presented an alternative epistemology of practice in which people gain knowledge through experience.

Schön's (1987) theory suggested people learn in two different ways. Firstly, people gain knowledge through what he called reflection in action. Reflection in action, also known as thinking on your feet, involves developing new understandings to inform our actions in the situation that is unfolding. Schön suggested that when individuals go about the spontaneous, intuitive performance of actions of everyday life, they demonstrate specific knowledge. However, often this knowledge cannot be articulated; individuals cannot say what they know, they do what they know (i.e., knowledge is in action). For example, a child will be able to coordinate the multiple bodily movements involved in throwing a ball and judge the distance of a target; however, it is unlikely that they would be able to articulate how they did this. Similarly, people learn life skills by being in a sporting environment but they may not be able to articulate which skills they learnt or how they learned them.

An individual restructures his/her understanding of the situation and invents new strategies of action. Individuals then try out new strategies as and when similar situations present themselves. Overall, reflection in action is non-cognitive knowing (Van Manen, 1999) in which knowledge resides in the actions that are lived and experienced by individuals. As such, if young people have been involved in organized sport programs it is reasonable to conclude that they will have been exposed to a range of skill building experiences. However, young people may be unaware of knowledge in action that they have acquired during their sporting experiences (i.e., the life skills they have learnt and the applicability of these skills across domains).

In order to highlight what people learn, and to prevent individuals becoming narrow, repetitive, conservative, and unreflective, they need to employ another type of reflection. People can use reflection on action to explore why we acted as we did, what was happening in a situation and why, what we have learned, and how we can use this knowledge in the future. The outcome of reflection on action is a repertoire of thoughts and ideas, based on successful response strategies, and outcomes that one can draw upon when confronted with new scenarios. Schön (1987) posited that this repertoire is central to reflective thought. Specifically, when an individual makes sense of a situation they perceive to be unique they relate it to previous experiences. The familiar experience (i.e., sport) functions as a precedent, a metaphor, or an exemplar for the unfamiliar one (i.e., a non-sport life domain) therefore allowing one to function when in unfamiliar scenarios (Schön, 1987). The true value of reflection on action is revealed when questions cannot be answered in the present. The process of reflection on action after an event allows us to approach these questions.

Reflection on action can take the form of retrospective reflection on action, in which an individual thinks back to experiences, and anticipatory reflection on action, in which an individual anticipates what future scenarios they may face. Specific strategies to engage in reflection on action include journaling, group discussions, and one-to-one meetings. It is important to have structured reflection so that individuals ask appropriate questions to ensure the reflection goes somewhere meaningful.

The individual is fully implicated in the phenomena that he or she documents. Reflective practitioners need to understand that what one sees in the self-examination process might be distorted (as is one's image in a mirror). Therefore, an individual cannot accomplish reflection on his or her own. Participants in life skills programs need the guidance of a "critical friend" to help guide the reflective process and to facilitate critical reflection.

Bourdieu (1990) argued a similar process in the learning of skills that orient the action of people in the social world. Bourdieu introduced the concept of habitus, as lasting, acquired schemes of perception, thought, and action that become unconscious and spontaneous. According to Bourdieu, an individual develops dispositions in response to the conditions he/she encounters in the field (i.e., in sport). Individuals' practice is always socially situated and therefore is specific to the field in which one is acting, at that moment. Bourdieu (1996) stated that persons are incarnations of the requirements of a given field. Thus, the requirements of sporting contexts will reflect the skills that young people learn. For example, a team sport like football will require young people to learn teamwork skills whereas sports like distance running, may result in the development of diligence and independence.

From an experiential learning / habitus perspective, researchers can explain the efficacy of a life skills program in terms of how life skills programs comprise, or form part of, a crystalizing experience. Walters and Gardner (1984) described crystallizing experiences in the context of talent and giftedness. Walters and Gardner defined a crystalizing experience as "the overt reaction of an individual to some quality or feature of a domain: the reaction yields an immediate but also a long term change in that individuals concept of the domain, his performance in it, and his view of himself" (p. 309). Crystalizing experiences may be initial experiences or refining experiences. Initial experiences are those that occur early in life and signal a general affinity between an individual and some large-scale domain (e.g., the initiation into sport). Refining experiences are those that occur later in life and comprise a discovery of a "particular instrument, style or approach within a field to which he or she is especially attuned" (Walters & Gardner, 1984, p. 309). These experiences are not entirely necessary in terms of actualizing thriving; however, they may be useful for explaining how individuals transfer skills from a life skills program to another life domain.

Jones, Lavallee, and Tod (2011b) suggested the sport provides young people with a range of developmental experiences, however, young people may not understand, or believe, that they possess skill. It is possible that through life skills programs, young people encounter materials (e.g., trained persons, engaging tasks) that activate latent skills. It is possible that through a life skills program, an individual could change how they choose to think about life and how they think about themselves. With the principle of latent skills in mind, Jones et al (2011b) developed a life skills program to help young people increase the awareness of the skills they had developed through sport, which they may not have known about. Jones and colleagues developed the Enhancement of Leadership, Intercommunication, Teamwork and Excellence (ELITE) life skills program as a method of increasing perceived use of life skills through reflective practice. Jones et al. developed the ELITE intervention as an eight-week life skills program that had the broad aim of increasing participants' self-awareness of perceived life skills, which participants had developed through sport experiences. Walters and Gardner (1984, p. 309) stated that "only retrospectively, after the individuals behavior in the post crystalizing period has been observed, is it possible to single out an experience as having crystalizing ensuing activities." It was Jones et al.'s (2011b) assumption that young people did learn life skills through sport, but the individual may not have been aware of these skills. Moreover, the individual may have been aware of the skills but could not articulate or understand that the skills was transferable. In essence, Jones and colleagues (2011b) could have suggested that youth sport experiences have crystalizing ensuing activities and therefore reflection on action was warranted.

Based on the results of Jones and Lavallee (2009), Jones et al. (2011b) decided to target communication skills and organization skills in the ELITE life skills program. Jones and Lavallee (2009) conducted a series of focus groups with athletes (aged 15–22 years), coaches, and experts in youth sport and sport psychology. The participants of Jones and Lavallee's (2009) focus groups believed that communication and organization skills were the most important life skills for British adolescent athletes to develop. Jones and Lavallee (2009) described communication skills and organization skills as umbrella terms for groups of life skills and they stated that these skills are important for positive development (e.g., Dworkin, Larson, & Hansen, 2003; Hansen et al., 2003; Larson, 2000; Larson, Hansen, & Moneta, 2006).

Jones and colleagues (2011b) designed the ELITE program as a two phase, eight-week life skills program that comprised one phase of communication skill reflections and one phase of organization skill reflection. Each phase included one week of reflecting on skills used in competition, one week of reflecting on skills used in training, one week of planning for anticipated scenarios where life skills might be needed, and one week of practicing skills ready for aforementioned scenarios. After each session, Jones and colleagues asked participants to complete a 28-item measure of perceived life skills. Each graph showed the progression of perceived life skill use in a baseline period, where no intervention was present, followed by the two phases of the ELITE and two weeks of a follow up period. Once the intervention was completed, the participants also completed a social validity interview to examine the extent to which the participants felt that the ELITE procedures were acceptable, the extent to which communication and organization skills were important to the participants, and whether the participants were satisfied with the program.

Results revealed that the process of thinking about previous sport experiences and planning for similar experiences in the future could increase perceived use of communication and organization skills and that participants valued the intervention and they enjoyed the sessions. Interestingly, the biggest improvement were seen in the female tennis players, compared with the male field hockey players, which may suggest a potential gender and or sport difference in how life skills are learned. The problem with Jones and colleagues (2011b) ELITE life skills program is that the authors did not directly measure the transferability of skills across life domains. Given the central theme of transferability in the conceptualization of life skills, future researchers need to establish whether programs such as the ELITE life skills program and other refining crystalizing experiences are transformative (i.e., the skills transfer across life domains).

Transfer of Life Skills as a Threshold Concept

Transferability of life skills from one life domain to another, or several other life domains, is a critical aspect of program efficacy that researchers often overlook. Gould and Carson noted that many practitioners base their life skills programs on the assumption that life skills carry over into different life domains; however, there is little evidence to substantiate this assumption. If an individual does not transfer a skill, that skill is arguably not a life skill (Jones, 2012), consequently, transferability is a core concept that research and practitioners need to carefully consider when developing life skills programs. Scholars have forwarded several theories regarding life skills transfer. For example, Danish, Petitpas, and Hale (1993) stated one of the barriers to skill transfer may be that athletes are not aware of the skills they have developed through sport that are transferable to other areas of life. Danish and colleagues suggested several factors and characteristics that can encourage transfer of skills. People could transfer life skills to other life domains if they increase their awareness of the skills they have acquired through their experiences in sport, knowledge of how and in what context they learned skills and awareness that these skills are valued in other life domains and that they can apply these skills in other life domains. Mayocchi and Hanrahan (2000) also suggested self-awareness was a critical element in developing life skills. Although, like Danish and colleagues, Mayocchi and Hanrahan do not guarantee transfer of life skills, they drew upon research from organizational psychology and sport psychology to develop a set of methods to enhance skill transfer. They identified individual characteristics including perceived value and level of skills awareness, motivation, and enthusiasm, and self-efficacy in moderating skills transfer. In order to facilitate transfer they also suggested athletes could be encouraged to increase their awareness of the skills they possess, when to use skills, and how they learned skills. Furthermore, program leaders could provide athletes with feedback about their attempts to transfer skills and help in developing action plans for use of skills in the future. Mayocchi and Hanrahan concluded:

> Without an understanding of the value of the types of skills that they possess, and an awareness of when certain skills may be applicable in different settings it is likely that skill transfer will occur by chance or unintentionally, if at all. Therefore, the challenge is to help athletes realize and identify what skills they have developed through sport so that, where relevant, these skills will be applied in different settings (p. 101).

The concept of transferability, and the process of transferability, may provide an example of what Meyer and Land (2003) coined threshold concepts. A threshold concept can open up a new and previously inaccessible way of thinking about something and may represent a transformed way of understanding or interpreting phenomena. Once an individual comprehends a threshold concept, they could be opened up to a transformed view of subject matter or even worldview (Meyer & Land, 2003). The understanding of transfer could open the individual up to a new understanding of where people can use their skills in the rest of their life.

It is our contention that life skills programs could provide the basis for a conceptual gateway that could be transformative and irreversible. This gateway can open up young people to the possibility of skills transfer outside of the life skills program. Once program participants understand that transfer could occur, and how transfer occurs, they can begin the process of skill transfer without the need for another life skills program. From this perspective, the outcome of a life skill program could be a conceptual space where the program participant looks at their life experience through a different lens. Whether a young person steps into a new conceptual space could be reflected by a shift in language used in relation to new understandings of life skill possibilities (Meyer & Land, 2005). Consequently, and in line with Gould and Carson's suggestion to improve methods of measurement, future researchers may want to consider life skills participants' dialogues with program leaders and peers as an indicator of positive development.

Are Life Skills Additive or Multiplicative?

Social environment and direct utility factors may work individually or interact to explain why developing life skills enhance child development. However, too often researchers have failed to identify explanations for how life skills may function to improve a young person's life and well-being. Doing so should be a high priority for future investigators.

(Gould & Carson, p. 67, 2008)

Simonton (1999) proposed a model of talent development on a belief that components of talent (e.g., height, hand eye coordination, general intelligence) should be multiplied together in order to understand an individual's talent potential (i.e., talent as a latent variable). Before the publication of this paper, Simonton noted that other researchers had predicted an individual's talent potential by adding up the number of talent components they possess. Simonton labeled these two models multiplicative and additive models of talent development, respectively. Although, Simonton discussed his emergenic model in the context of talent development, we believe it could be possible to use some of the same principles when discussing thriving and optimal human functioning.

Based on an additive model, thriving and optimal functioning constitutes a linear sum of contributing components (e.g., separate life skills). For example, for an individual to thrive they need to accumulate a number of life skills in adequate amounts. The more skills a person possesses, the more they will thrive. The majority of positive youth development theories are predicated on this principle. For example, Benson (2007) sated that the 40 developmental assets theory is based on a "more assets are better" hypothesis, or a vertical pile up, or stacking, of assets. According to Benson, accumulated assets generalize into multiple forms of behavior, which may include prevention of high-risk behavior and/or enhancement of optimal functioning. Lerner's 5Cs model is also based on an additive hypothesis. The more Cs the better, the higher each individual scores on each C, the better. From an additive model, it is possible for an individual to achieve optimal human functioning even if they have no capacity in just one of the essential elements. From an additive perspective, practitioners and scholars could measure optimal functioning potential via the sum of functioning / thriving components. For example, we could use Lerner's 5Cs as thriving components, where each C (caring, competence, confidence, character, connection) represents one possible thriving component. If we use a hypothetical scoring system where we score each C on a 6-point Likert scale (e.g. 0-5), a given individual can obtain a thriving potential score of 0-25. For example, if an individual scores high on caring (score =5/5), connection (score =5/5), confidence (score =5/5) and competence (score =5/5), but she does not demonstrate any character (score 0/5) thriving potential could be calculated as 20/25, which for arguments sake is an above average score. Readers may notice that the range of possible scores is low (0-25) and so additive models may have reduced predictive accuracy.

Alternatively, a multiplicative model of thriving is predicated on multiplication of core components (e.g., life skills). From this perspective, for an individual to achieve optimal functioning, they need to accumulate life skills in combination. If skills are absent, a person can still function successfully but might not function optimally within that domain. A multiplicative model of optimal functioning requires an interactive, bidirectional interplay of specific life skills, without this, thriving is not just diminished but fails to gather traction. The key difference between multiplicative and additive perspectives is evident when an individual does not possess a core component. In an additive model, an individual can circumvent one component with other components and in the absence of one core component, the individual can still achieve a high thriving potential. In a multiplicative model, if an individual is missing one core components thriving may not occur. By using the same 5Cs example, if our individual scores high on caring (score =5/5), connection (score =5/5), confidence (score =5/5) and competence (score =5/5) but she does not demonstrate any character (score 0/5) her thriving potential is 0/3125 (because we calculate thriving potential by multiplying each core component by the others: 5x5x5x5x0). From an additive model, this individual has an above average score but from multiplicative model, she has a very low, below average score. If the same person improves and can generate a score of 1/5 for character, she would move from 0 to 625/3125 (i.e., 5x5x5x5x1).

If someone has no capacity for one of the essential components, then that person may not be able to display any thriving potential (assuming that thriving and talent are conceptually similar: cf, Simonton, 1999). Readers could also note the differences in the range of possible scores between an additive and a multiplicative model of thriving. In our hypothetical additive model there is a range of 0-25 whereas in our multiplicative model a range of 0-3125 may contribute to higher predictive accuracy.

It is important for researchers to consider the differences between additive and multiplicative models of thriving because the outcome of a life skills program could be positive from one perspective but not the other.

Although it is not our intention to provide definitive answers to the questions of additive or multiplicative models of thriving, we do encourage researchers to consider this problem, to make personal biases clear when describing the program, and to adapt life skills programs based on varied epistemological perspectives of life skill development.

If this area is to progress towards greater predictive accuracy then researchers need to be more specific regarding what behavior, which assets, and how these assets interact with one another, within the individual and their social milieu. A 'more is better' approach could be too simplistic.

Conclusion

The purpose of this chapter was to provide an overview of what we consider to be some important concepts and debates in the current life skill literature and to discuss possible reasons why life skill programs are effective in facilitating optimal human functioning. We hope that it is evident that the development of life skills is a worthy venture, however the best way to promote life skills developments is unclear.

A major problem with the extant literature is a lack of robust studies that test the efficacy of life skills programs and the transferability of life skills from one life domain to another. Moreover, there is a lack of procedural detail that means independent researchers cannot repeat the life skills program.

In our opinion, the most promising theoretical explanation for the efficacy of life skill programs lies in the social interactions research.

We believe that studies of coach education, peer interaction, and parent influences provide researchers with a solid basis upon which to investigate the process of program efficacy. Future researchers and practitioners may wish to manipulate different modes of social interaction to examine which social agent, or combination of agents, augment the development of life skills.

We believe that research from talent development, education, and coaching can help life skills program leaders to develop better life skills programs. We hope that discussion of crystalizing experiences, threshold concepts, and vertical stacking vs. multiplicative models of life skills provide the reader with food for thought and we encourage debate amongst scholars and practitioners on these ideas.

REFERENCES

Barnett, N. P., Smoll, F. L., & Smith, R. E. (1992). Effects of enhancing coach-athlete relationships on youth sport attrition. *The Sport Psychologist, 6,* 111-127.

Benson, P. L. (2007). Developmental assets: An overview of theory, research, and practice. In R. K. Silbereisen & R. M. Lerner (Eds.), *Approaches to positive youth development* (pp. 33-58), London, UK: Sage.

Bourdieu, P. (1990). *The logic of practice*. Cambridge, UK: Polity Press.

Bourdieu, P. (1996). *The state nobility*. Cambridge, UK: Polity Press.

Camiré, M., Trudel, P., & Forneris, T. (2012). Coaching and transferring life skills: Philosophies and strategies used by model high school coaches. *The Sport Psychologist, 26*, 243-260.

Catalano, R. F., Berglund, M. L., Ryan, J. A. M., Lonczak, H. S., & Hawkins, J. D. (1998). *Positive youth development in the United States: Research findings on evaluations of youth development programs*. Washington, DC: US Department of Health and Human Services.

Coatsworth, J. D., & Conroy, D. E. (2006). Enhancing the self-esteem of youth swimmers through coach training: Gender and age effects. *Psychology of Sport and Exercise, 7,* 173-192.

Conroy, D. E., & Coatsworth, J. D. (2006). Coach training as a strategy for promoting youth social development. *The Sport Psychologist, 20,* 128-144.

Côté, J. (1999). The influence of the family in the development of talent in sport. *The Sport Psychologist, 13,* 395-417.

Côté, J., & Hay, J. (2002). Children's involvement in sport: A developmental perspective. In J. M. Silva & D. E. Stevens (Eds.), *Psychological foundations of sport* (pp. 484-502). Boston, MA: Allyn & Bacon.

Crisp, S. (1998). International models of best practice in wilderness and adventure therapy. In C. Itin (Ed.). *Exploring the boundaries of adventure therapy: International perspectives* (pp. 56-74). Boulder, CO: Association for Experiential Education.

Csikszentmihalyi, M., & Rathunde, K. (1998). The development of the person: An experiential perspective on the ontogenesis of psychological complexity. In W. Damon & R. M. Lerner (Eds in Chief) &.) & R. M Lerner (Vol. Ed.), *Handbook of Child Psychology: Vol.1. Theoretical models of human development* (5th ed. pp. 635-684). New York, NY: Wiley.

Danish, S. J., Nellen, V. C., & Owens, S. S. (1996). Teaching life skills through sport: Community-based programs for adolescents. In J. L. Van Raalte & B. W. Brewer (Eds.), *Exploring sport and exercise psychology* (pp. 205-225). Washington DC: American Psychological Association.

Danish, S. J., Petitpas, A. J., & Hale, B. D. (1993). Life development intervention for athletes: Life skills through sports. *The Counseling Psychologist, (Major contribution) 21,* 352-385.

Dworkin, J. B., Larson, R. W., & Hansen, D. (2003). Adolescents' accounts of growth experiences in youth activities. *Journal of Youth and Adolescence, 32,* 17-26.

Eccles, J. S., Barber, B. L., Stone, M., & Hunt, J. (2003). Extracurricular activities and adolescent development. *Journal of Social Issues, 59,* 865-889.

Fraser-Thomas, J. L., Côté, J., & Deakin, J. (2005). Youth sport programs: An avenue to foster positive youth development. *Physical Education and Sport Pedagogy, 10,* 19-40.

Galton, F. (1869). *Hereditary genius.* London, UK: Macmillan and Company.

Gould, D., & Carson, S. (2008). Life skills development through sport: Current status and future directions. *International review of sport and exercise psychology, 1,* 58-78.

Gould, D., Chung, Y., Smith, P., & White, W. (2006). Future directions in coaching life skills: Understanding high school coaches' views and needs. *Athletic Insight, 8.* Retrieved March 1, 2013, from http://www.athleticinsight.com/Vol8Iss3/CoachingLifeSkills.htm.

Gould, D., Collins, K., Lauer, L., & Chung, Y. (2005). Coaching life skills: A working model. *Sport and Exercise Psychology Review, 2,* 4-12.

Hansen, D. M., Larson, R. W., & Dworkin, J. B. (2003). What adolescents learn in organized youth activities: A survey of self-reported developmental experiences. *Journal of Research on Adolescence, 13,* 25-55.

Hellison, D. (2003). *Teaching responsibility through physical activity* (2nd ed.). Champaign, IL: Human Kinetics.

Jelicic, H., Theokas, C., Phelps, E., & Lerner, R. M. (2007). Conceptualizing and measuring the context within person ←→ context models of human development: Implications for theory, research, and application. In T. D. Little, J. A. Bovaird & N. A. Card. (Eds.), *Modeling ecological and contextual effects in longitudinal studies of human development* (pp. 437-457). Mahwah, NJ: Erlbaum.

Jones, M. I. (2012). Developing life skills in athletes. In S. Hanton & S. D. Mellalieu (Eds.), *Professional practice in sport psychology: A review* (pp. 249-272). London, UK: Routledge.

Jones, M. I., Dunn, J. G. H., Holt, N. L., Sullivan, P. J., & Bloom, G. A. (2011a). Exploring the '5Cs' of positive youth development in sport. *Journal of Sport Behavior, 34,* 250-267.

Jones, M. I., & Lavallee, D. (2009). Exploring the life skills needs of adolescent athletes. *Psychology of Sport and Exercise, 10,* 159-167.

Jones, M. I., Lavallee, D., & Tod, D. (2011b). Developing communication and organization skills: The ELITE life skills reflective practice program. *The Sport Psychologist, 25,* 159-176.

Larson, R. W. (2000). Toward a psychology of positive youth development. *American Psychologist, 55,* 170-183.

Larson, R. W., Hansen, D., & Moneta, G. (2006). Differing profiles of developmental experiences across types of organized youth activities. *Developmental Psychology, 42,* 849-863.

Lerner, R. M. (2004). *Liberty: Thriving and civic engagement among American youth.* Thousand Oaks, CA: Sage Publications.

Lerner, R. M. (2005, September). *Promoting positive youth development: Theoretical and empirical bases.* White paper prepared for the Workshop on the Science of Adolescent

Health and Development, National Research Council/Institute of Medicine. Washington D.C.: National Academies of Science.

Lerner, R. M., Almerigi, J. B., Theokas, C., & Lerner, J. V. (2005). Positive youth development: A view of the issues. *Journal of Early Adolescence, 25,* 10-16.

Lerner, R. M., Lerner, J. V., Almerigi, J., Theokas, C., Phelps, E., Naudeau, S., et al. (2006). Toward a new vision and vocabulary about adolescence: Theoretical and empirical bases of a "positive youth development" perspective. In L. Balter, & C. S. Tamis-LeMonda (Eds.), *Child psychology: A handbook of contemporary issues* (pp. 445-469). New York, NY: Taylor & Francis.

Mandela, N. (1995). *A long walk to freedom.* London, UK: Abacus.

Mayocchi, L., & Hanrahan, S. J. (2000). Transferable skills for career change. In D. Lavallee & P. Wylleman (Eds.), *Career transitions in sport: International perspectives* (pp. 95-110). Morgantown, WV: Fitness Information Technology.

McCallister, S. G., Blinde, E. M., & Weiss, W. M. (2000). Teaching values and implementing philosophies: Dilemmas of the coach. *Physical Educator, 57,* 35-45.

McCloy, C. (1930). Character building through physical education. *Research Quarterly, 1,* 41-61.

Meyer, J. H. F., & Land, R. (2003). Threshold concepts and troublesome knowledge: Linkages to ways of thinking and practising within the disciplines. In C. Rust (Ed.), *Improving student learning: improving student learning theory and practice – ten years on* (pp. 1-16). Oxford, UK: Oxford Centre for Staff and Learning Development.

Meyer, J. H. F., & Land, R. (2005). Threshold concepts and troublesome knowledge (2): Epistemological considerations and a conceptual framework for teaching and learning. *Higher education, 49,* 373-388.

Miller, P. S., & Kerr, G. A. (2002). Conceptualizing excellence: Past, present, and future. *Journal of Applied Sport Psychology, 14,* 140-153.

National Research Council and Institute of Medicine (2002*). Community programs to promote youth development: Committee on community-level programs for youth.* Board of Children, Youth, and Families, Division of Behavioral and Social Sciences and Education. Washington DC: National Academy Press.

Ogilvie, B. C., & Tutko, A. T. (1971). If you want to build character, try something else. *Psychology Today, 5,* 60-63.

Petitpas, A. J., Cornelius, A., & Van Raalte, J. (2008). Youth development through sport: It's all about the relationships. In N. L. Holt (Ed.), *Positive youth development through sport* (pp. 61-71). New York: Routledge.

Petitpas, A. J., Cornelius, A. E., Van Raalte, J. L., & Jones, T. (2005). A framework for planning youth sport programs that foster psychosocial development. *The Sport Psychologist, 19,* 63-80.

Pope John Paul II. (2000). Address of John Paul II to the international convention on the theme: *During the time of the jubilee: The face and soul of sport.* Retrieved on 19 March, 2013 from http://www.vatican.va/holy_father/john_paul_ii/speeches/documents/hf_jp-ii_spe_20001028_jubilsport_en.html

Rhodes, J. E. (2004). The critical ingredient: Caring youth –staff relationships in after school settings. *New Directions for Youth Development, 10,* 145-161.

Robert, J. S., Hall, B. K., & Olson, W. M. (2003). Bridging the gap between developmental systems theory and evolutionary developmental biology. *BioEssays, 23,* 954-962.

Rogge, J. (2004). *IOC and UNAIDS join forces to engage sport community in fight against aids*. IOC Press Release, 1 June.

Roth, J. L., & Brooks-Gunn, J. (2003). What exactly is a youth development program? Answers from research and practice. *Applied Developmental Science*, *7*, 94-111.

Schön, D. (1987). *Educating the reflective practitioner*. San Francisco: Jossey-Bass.

Shabani, K., Khatib, M., & Ebadi, S. (2010). Vygotsky's zone of proximal development: Instructional implications and teachers' professional development. *English language teaching*, *3*, 237-248.

Simonton, D. K. (1999). Talent and its development: An emergenic and epigenetic model. *Psychological Review*, *106*, 435.

Smith, R. E., Smoll, F. L., & Barnett, N. P. (1995). Reduction of children's sport performance anxiety through social support and stress-reduction training for coaches. *Journal of Applied Developmental Psychology, 16,* 125-142.

Smith, R. E., Smoll, F. L., & Curtis, B. (1979). Coach effectiveness training: A cognitive behavioral approach to enhancing relationship skills in youth sport coaches. *Journal of Sport Psychology, 1,* 59-75.

Smoll, F. L., & Smith, R. E. (1984). Leadership research in youth sports. In J. M. Silva & R. S. Weinberg (Eds.), *Psychological foundations of sport* (pp. 371-386). Champaign, IL: Human Kinetics.

Smoll, F. L., Smith, R. E., Barnett, N. P., & Everett, J. J. (1993). Enhancement of children's self-esteem through social support training for youth sport coaches. *Journal of Applied Psychology, 78,* 602-610.

UNICEF (2003). *Definition of terms*. Retrieved April 12, 2013, from http://www.unicef.org/lifeskills/index_7308.html.

Van Manen, M. (1999). The practice of practice. In M. Lange, J. Olson, H. Hansen, & W. Bÿnder (Eds.), *Changing schools/changing practices: Perspectives on educational reform and teacher professionalism*. Luvain, Belgium: Garant. Retrieved August 2, 2007 from http://www.phenomenologyonline.com/max/articles/practice.html.

Vygotsky, L. S. (1962). *Thought and language*. MIT press.

Vygotsky, L. S. (1978). *Mind in society: The development of higher psychological processes*. Cambridge, MA: Harvard University Press.

Walters, J., & Gardner, H. (1984). The crystallizing experience: Discovering an intellectual. In R. Sternberg &W. J. Davidson (Eds.), *Conceptions of Giftedness* (pp. 306-331). New York: Cambridge University Press.

Weiss, M. R., & Gill, D. L. (2005). What goes around comes around: Re-emerging themes in sport and exercise psychology. *Research Quarterly for Exercise and Sport, 76*, S71-S87.

World Health Organization. (1999). *Partners in life skills education*. Geneva, Switzerland: World Health Organization, Department of Mental Health.

In: Positive Human Functioning ... Volume 2 ISBN: 978-1-62948-973-5
Editors: A. R. Gomes, R. Resende and A. Albuquerque © 2014 Nova Science Publishers, Inc.

Chapter 3

POSITIVE HUMAN DEVELOPMENT: TEACHING POSITIVE LIVING SKILLS TO CHILDREN AND YOUTH

Terry Orlick
School of Human Kinetics, University of Ottawa, Ottawa, Canada

ABSTRACT

In this chapter, Terry Orlick highlights the urgent need to integrate Positive Living Skills initiatives within our families, schools, homes and communities worldwide. A general introduction to Positive Living Skills is presented, the multiple benefits of Positive Living Skills Educational Initiatives are discussed and the tools to begin implementing these positive life enhancement initiatives are shared. The author draws attention to the critical importance of beginning these positive initiatives with children and youth right now. The advantages of positive living skills are weighed against the consequences of negative living skills. The author emphasizes that the road to a higher level humanity and a healthier and more compassionate world can begin right now by teaching children and youth Positive Living Skills which can continue to be nurtured, improved and refined throughout their lives.

INTRODUCTION

The extent to which we nurture Positive Human Development will dictate the future of humanity on our planet. If we are serious about helping Positive Human Interaction to flourish on our planet, we need to make a personal and global commitment to teach and nurture Positive Living Skills to children and youth. The best way to eliminate most negativity in schools, homes, neighborhoods, playgrounds, communities, governments and places of work is to stop negative actions and negative interactions before they start by providing positive alternatives. We can accomplish this goal by teaching children and youth Positive Living Skills at an early age in their homes, schools, playgrounds and neighborhoods. It is easier to prevent fires before they start than to try to put out raging fires, as they burn down everything in their path—houses, forests, jungles, humans, animals and communities. In the same way, it is easier to prevent negative human problems before they start than to try to fix those problems after they have started. The unfortunate reality on our planet is that there are many millions of negative and destructive people who do their best to make the lives of other people miserable. Virtually all people problems, relationships problems, anger problems, abuse problems, and bullying problems are directly related to people being negative, disrespectful, or inconsiderate to others. They do this by putting other people down, being disrespectful, hurting, bullying, humiliating, degrading others, and in some cases by torturing or killing other human beings physically or emotionally. This kind of negativity can surface in many contexts, for example, in schools, homes, families, relationships, villages, neighborhoods, communities, cities, governments, places of work, playgrounds, and sporting events. This kind of negativity is also spread across various forms of mass media where brutal violence and negativity is often depicted graphically (i.e. in television shows, news reports, movies, and throughout the Internet).

In order to nurture a higher level of humanity in the homes, schools, and communities throughout our planet, we need to introduce Positive Living Skills Educational Programs that will help all children and youth to learn and grow in more positive and compassionate ways. This is why I created the Positive Living Skills Educational Program – to help both teachers and parents enhance and nurture Positive Human Development within their children. The Positive Living Skills Educational Program can help us to begin this nurturing and positive growth Right Now. The best place to begin the journey to improved global humanity is with the children and youth in our schools, homes, and communities in every corner of our world.

Why Do People Hurt Other People?

Those who hurt, bully, put down, degrade or destroy others in physical, mental, social and emotional ways usually do so because (1) they are copying the negative actions of others, or (2) they have never been taught how to behave, act, live, or interact in positive and life enhancing ways. In addition, many children, youth and adults who are negative towards others also feel negative or insecure about themselves. If we can help these individuals to look for and see value, hope, positive possibilities and positive qualities within themselves and within others, they will begin to develop a more positive life perspective, and engage with others in more compassionate and empathetic ways.

People who are negative are people who have failed to learn how to be positive. The consequences of learning to become negative as opposed to positive can be extreme and endure over an entire lifetime. In the beginning and the end, learning to be positive (as opposed to negative) makes the difference between (1) finding and embracing simple uplifting experiences, simple joys and Highlights every day, and not being able to find or embrace these daily uplifting experiences; (2) being physically, mentally and emotionally happy, and being physically, mentally and emotionally discontent; and (3) being focused in life enhancing ways, and being focused in negative and energy draining ways.

Fortunately, we have a choice with respect to how we educate our children and youth. If we introduce Positive Living Skills education programs to children at an early age, we can help all children and youth learn how to live in more positive, focused, and fully connected ways. In turn, this will lead to living healthier, happier, more respectful, more joyful, more focused, and more meaningful lives. It is very easy to teach most children how to find and embrace simple uplifting experiences (Highlights or simple joys) in every day, and how to focus in more fully connected ways (Orlick, 2011).

There are many good reasons to begin teaching Positive Living Skills to children at any early age. It is much easier to prevent both environmental pollution and negative human development pollution before it starts. If we wait until negativity has been engrained in children's minds, the challenge of positive change becomes much more difficult.

We can enhance the lives of children, teenagers, students, families, athletes, teams, performers, parents, teachers and others by replacing negative ways of being with positive ways of being. We can begin this educational journey right now by introducing the Positive Living Skills Educational Initiative. All that is required is that we make a personal and professional commitment to teach children and youth essential Positive Living Skills that they can use in every facet of their lives.

THE ROOTS OF POSITIVE CHANGE

As a society, we invest large amounts of time, money, and energy to teach children academic skills – for example, how to read and write, how to figure out math problems, and learn about many other subjects. We do everything we can to ensure that children learn to read and write. We encourage them to practice their reading and writing skills, help them work on improving their reading and writing skills and often continue to help them develop their reading and writing skills over the course of their lives. We clearly understand that if we want children to learn how to read and write, we have to teach them how to read and write and provide them with opportunities to practice and improve these skills over the course of many years. We do not simply tell children to read or write and expect them to learn and perfect these skills on their own. We make a conscious and deliberate decision to help them learn the essential skills that are required for literacy and we act in positive and concrete ways to make this happen.

If we want to ensure that children, youth, and adults learn how to live their lives in positive, focused and life enhancing ways, we need to teach them how to do this. We need to develop and implement a Positive Living Skills curriculum so that children, youth and adults will learn essential skills that will empower them to be better people, better communicators, better learners, better performers, and positive contributors to a better world.

A well designed and well implemented Positive Living Skills curriculum will also reduce and, in many cases, eliminate the rising tide of unnecessary bullying, negativity, conflict, violence, abuse, and negative human interaction problems that we witness every day across the world. To live the positive lives that we are all capable of living, we desperately need to implement a Global Positive Living Action Plan to teach and nurture Positive Living Skills to children and youth in all parts of the world.

Teachers, parents, coaches, students and other supportive people need to become an integral part of this Positive Human Development Action Team. Opportunities for Positive Living Skills education become possible whenever we are interacting, playing or working with young people in any context, for example at school, at home, in the community, when children are engaged in all kinds of interactions: free play, games, sports, physical activity, or performing arts (dancing, acting, singing, and making music). Teachers, coaches, parents, siblings, teammates, friends can engage themselves in meaningful positive actions to help other children, students, athletes, educators and performers to learn, develop, and refine essential skills that are required for ongoing positive living, positive learning, positive interaction, and positive performances. This will help virtually all children, students, learners, players, and performers to learn the great and numerous benefits of positive living and in turn, these people will help others learn similar essential skills for positive growth. We need to act on our positive intentions and support others in acting on their positive intentions. We cannot just leave it to chance! As leaving it to chance alone is not working very well in our world.

We need the support of as many people as possible to jump-start positive change – children, students, parents, teachers, educators, counselors, coaches, principals, professors, researchers, consultants, school boards, media outlets, companies and members of the community who are fully committed to positive human development. In essence, we need positive action-based planning. We need many avenues to implement positive plans, such as through policy and curriculum development. We need the collective support of many caring people who will introduce and support positive educational initiatives.

As a result of my extensive applied work and research with Positive Living Skills, I believe they are the most essential skills that anyone can learn to enhance productive and connected focusing for positive living, learning, performance, and interactions that will impact on the overall quality of our lives. This has led me to ask myself and others the following question – *If Positive Living Skills Educational Initiatives can enhance positive human development and quality of life for all people, why are these initiatives absent in our schools, homes, and communities?*

Why are we not teaching and nurturing Positive Living Skills in meaningful and systematic ways with billions of children from every corner of the world? Why are we not working together as teachers, parents, educators and caring human beings to nurture more positive young people who will then create a better, more positive world and future for everyone?

Is negativity and an absence of compassion for other human beings something we should be concerned about? Is negative behavior, violence and inflicting harm (both physical and psychological) something we should try to prevent from happening? Is positive, fully connected focus and compassion something we should begin to teach and nurture at an early age?

I would like you to take a few moments to think about and write down your responses to the following questions:

1. WHY WE SHOULD: Why should we introduce positive living skills to all children in the world?
2. WHY WE CAN: Why can we introduce positive living skills to all children in the world?
3. HOW WE WILL: How will we introduce positive living skills to all children in the world?
4. POSITIVE STEPS YOU CAN TAKE RIGHT NOW: What positive steps can **you** take or what positive things can **you** do right now to begin to act on your positive intentions?

Anyone who cares about the quality of children's' lives - including parents, teachers and students studying to become teachers, principals, members of school boards, as well as Professors in teacher education programs - can help to ensure that children and youth are given opportunities to learn how to live, learn, perform and interact in positive and life enhancing ways. They simply have to support the introduction of Positive Living Skills educational programs in all school contexts at all levels.

The applied research we have done with Positive Living Skills in the school system has clearly shown that students in elementary school, junior high school, high school and university need and benefit greatly from learning, practicing, refining and living with Positive Living Skills on a daily basis. Students in all of our studies reported that their personal quality of life was enhanced in meaningful ways by learning, applying and living with Positive Living Skills. They also reported using these skills in their everyday lives at school, at home and in many other contexts including sport and physical activity settings.

If we fail to teach and nurture Positive Living Skills with children and youth in our homes and schools, the most essential lessons for living in positive, connected and compassionate ways is left totally to chance. Unfortunately, leaving Positive Living Skills education to chance has not been working very well in schools and communities throughout the world. The state of our world and the harmony of our own lives and relationships are dependent on what we focus on, how we live each day, how we approach, see, and interact with ourselves and with others. As parents, teachers, educators, leaders, school administrators, professors, researchers, university students, high school students, coaches, athletes, performers and compassionate people who care about children, youth and the future of our world, we need to step up and be the leaders for positive change. We need to invest more time, resources and positive energy on teaching children and youth how to become better people, better learners, and better performers. By doing so, we will teach young people to live with and project more positivity, joyfulness, support, happiness, focus and compassion. This will free them to grow into more positive, relaxed and less stressed human brings, who will know how to contribute to positive relationships, positive communities and a more positive global world. This is the overall goal of Positive Living Skills Education.

CHARTING A POSITIVE PATH

Presented below are the Three Wheels of Positive Living, which provide a framework for you to begin nurturing Positive Highlights, Fully Connected Focus and Personal Excellence. There are many Positive Living Skills that we need to learn to live our lives in positive, productive and compassionate ways. These essential Positive Living Skills are presented graphically below as the Three Wheels of Positive Living. The first wheel of Positive Living is the Wheel of Highlights, the second wheel is the Wheel of Focus, and the third wheel is the Wheel of Excellence.

A Positive and Fully Connected Focus drives each of these Wheels forward in positive and life enhancing ways. In fact, the core of all three wheels for Positive Human Development, Positive Human Performance and Positive Human Interaction is a Positive and Fully Connected Focus. A Positive and Fully Connected Focus empowers us to find and embrace more Highlights, to focus in more positive and connected ways, and to live, learn and perform closer to our true human potential. A Positive and Fully Connected Focus provides the power that drives the different spokes of each wheel forward in positive ways. You will only move forward in positive and meaningful directions with the help of a positive and fully connected focus.

The first wheel of Positive Living is the **Wheel of Highlights**, sometimes also referred to as the Wheel of Simple Joys (Orlick, 2011).

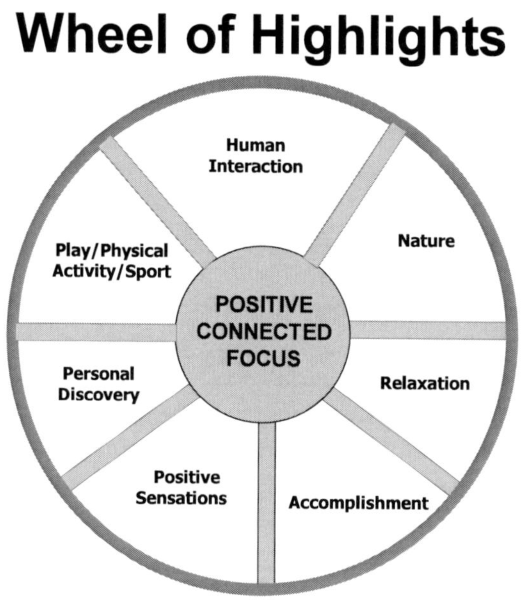

To find more Highlights in their life, we ask participants of all ages to look for and find simple Highlights everyday. We also ask participants to keep a Highlight Journal where at the end of the day they are encouraged to write down or record all the simple joys they found and experienced that day. Some students also take pictures of their Highlights or draw their Highlights and put them in their Highlight Journals. We ask participants to share some of their favorite Highlights with their classmates, teammates or family members on a regular basis. This kind of sharing promotes positive communication by encouraging everyone to focus on finding, sharing and listening to others' Highlights. Moreover, it allows participants to learn from their own journey of finding Highlights and recognize the possibility of experiencing new Highlights from their classmates, friends, teammates and family members. Sharing Highlights is a very important, positive and uplifting experience.

Seven Major Highlight Domains have surfaced from our extensive research on Highlights with children, youth and young adults:

- Human Interaction Highlights
- Nature Highlights
- Relaxation Highlights
- Personal Accomplishment Highlights
- Positive Sensations Highlights
- Personal Discovery Highlights and
- Play, Physical Activity & Sport Highlights

We encourage participants to embrace Highlights in as many different domains as possible every single day. Hunting for Highlights in different domains increases the joy and frequency of positive experiences that can be found in different domains everyday.

The second wheel of Positive Living is the **Wheel of Focus** (Orlick, 2011).

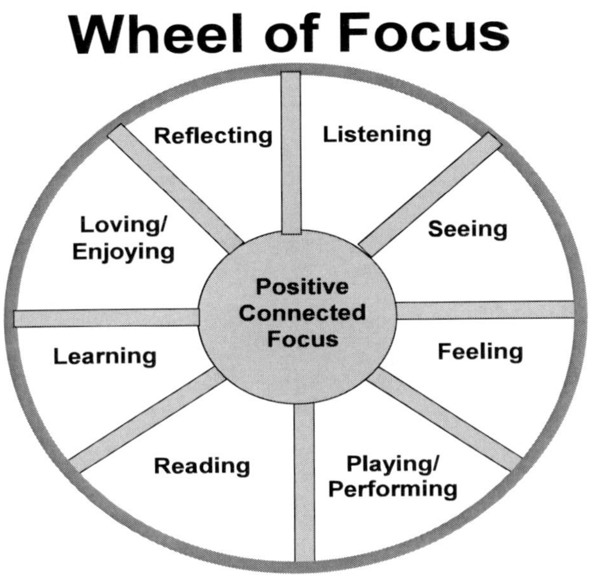

Our goal is to help children, students and people of all ages to focus in positive and fully connected ways in everything they do throughout their day. We want them to learn how to "be totally here mentally." Fundamentally, we ask the question, if you are "here" physically, why not also "be here" mentally? One of our goals is to ensure that children, youth and adults are given opportunities to practice being fully focused every day, because focus is a skill that can be learned, and practiced and always improved. It is also important to challenge children, youth, adults, students, learners, athletes, players, performers, partners to practice extending the time or duration for which they can sustain a positive and fully connected focus. How long can you actually "be here" positive and fully focused in this moment or context and "stay here" positive and fully focused in this moment or context?

It is a great advantage for people of all ages, living in all contexts, to learn how to enter and sustain a positive and fully connected focus. The following eight focus domains that are presented in the Wheel of Focus above include:

- Focused Listening
- Focused Seeing
- Focused Feeling
- Focused Playing / Performing
- Focused Reading
- Focused Learning
- Focused Loving / Enjoying
- Focused Reflection

All children, youth, adults, students, learners, performers, relationships, teachers, parents, family members, counselors, workers and leaders in all contexts at all levels can gain from enhancing the depth and duration of their positive and fully connected focus in each of the focus domains presented in the Wheel of Focus.

The third wheel of Positive Living is the **Wheel of Excellence** (Orlick, 2008).

Wheel of Excellence

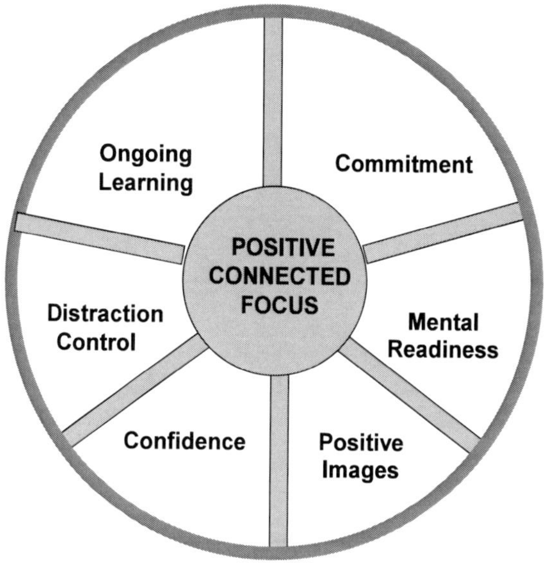

I use this Wheel extensively with anyone who wants to improve the quality of their learning, the quality of their performance and the consistency of their best performances. The Wheel of Excellence presents the Mental Skills that are required to perform at a high level in any performance domain.

- Commitment: How committed are you to practicing and perfecting the skills it takes to accomplish the goals that you set out to achieve, persevere through the ups and downs, learn from the positives, negatives, and ongoing challenges of your journey?
- Mental Readiness: Are you mentally ready and completely present and fully focused in the moment when you set out to do a specific task today, tomorrow, this month, this year, and in your lifetime?
- Positive Images: Do you imagine yourself performing your best and successfully accomplishing the goals that you set out to accomplish? Are you willing to continue to work on improving your positive imagery skills?

  Confidence: To what extent do you feel confident in yourself and confident in your ability to do what you really want to do? Are you willing to work on strengthening your confidence in positive ways that will help to accomplish what you want to accomplish?
- Distraction Control: How good are you at avoiding or letting go of unnecessary distractions that can interfere with your best performances? Can you stay fully

focused on doing what you want to do and refocus on what will help you perform to your true potential even when there are distractions around you?

- Ongoing Learning: Ongoing Learning and Acting in positive ways on the lessons learned from each interaction and performance scenario is essential for living, learning and performing to your true potential.

We encourage children, youth, performers and all other people to continue to draw positive focus lessons from each of their classes, preparation sessions, practices, performances, new experiences, and personal interactions. It is important to acknowledge the lessons that can be taken from negative, disappointing or unsuccessful situations, and often even more important to acknowledge, reflect and act on the lessons that can be learned from positive, uplifting and successful situations. Encourage children, youth and adults to continue to act on the lessons learned. This will help to ensure that everyone involved understands how to acknowledge, accept and grow from positive experiences and from less than best experiences. It is essential that you, your students and others with whom you live, work or play begin to act in positive ways on the focusing and refocusing lessons that can easily be taught, learned and nurtured every single day. This is the only way to ensure that you and others continue to grow and improve in positive, meaningful and sustainable life enhancing ways.

Acting on Positive Intentions

Now is the time for you and all other concerned citizens of the world to begin providing Positive Living Skills Educational opportunities in your schools, homes, neighborhoods, playgrounds, colleges, universities, sporting contexts and communities around the world. This is the only way that we can be sure that all children and youth are given positive opportunities to benefit from learning Positive Living Skills and embracing the simple joys and lessons learned from simply living their lives fully, respectfully and joyfully.

Parents, teachers, students, professors, researchers, writers, broadcasters, film makers and people of all ages, engaged in all kinds of work who would like to contribute to creating a better world, can begin by finding ways to use, teach, and promote positive living skills everyday. Any caring person at any age can begin sharing simple, positive, life-enhancing activities from my book *Positive Living Skills: Joy and Focus for Everyone* (Orlick, 2011). We can all encourage the continued use, improvement, and perfection of these life-enhancing skills over the course of our lives. By choosing to take this positive step forward we can help others understand and feel the vital importance of living their lives in positive and life enhancing ways. By simply choosing to take this step forward, we can also decide to be or become the best possible example of positive living for others to follow.

Bottom Line Reminders for Meaningful Positive Change

- **Be a Teacher:** Implement Positive Living Skills Programs by teaching Positive Living Skills to children and youth in your home, school or community.

- **Encourage New Teachers:** Teach courses on Quality Living to students in elementary school, junior high school, senior high school, college, and university who can then go out and teach Positive Living Skills to young people and others including business leaders, program directors at community centers, social development projects, camps, homes or any other potential learning context.
- **Move beyond Lip Service:** Remind children, teenagers, university students and adults with whom you work that thinking about what they want to do is not enough.
- **Only Action Counts:** When it comes to Positive Living, thinking is not enough. Even deciding is not enough. Teach, tell, and show those surrounding you that only action counts when it comes to positive and joyful living. Continue to remind others to act on their positive intentions in simple positive ways, every day.
- **Teach Through Example:** Be or become a positive living example for others to follow. Deeply integrate Positive Living Skills into your daily life.
- **Search for Positivity:** Find ways to be or become supportive, focused, relaxed, calm, helpful, compassionate and joyful in your own pursuits. Search for positivity in every facet of your life.
- **Help Others Understand the Benefits:** Help children, youth and adults to actually implement Positive Living Skills that will help them to live, learn, interact, relax, contribute and perform in more positive, compassionate and joyful ways over the course of their lives.
- **Remember and Reflect on the Benefits:** Remember that Positive Living Skills are the greatest gift we can give to children, youth and adults. It is only by teaching and nurturing Positive Ways of Being that we can raise the level of humanity in our own lives and in our world today and influence a better, happier and more humane global environment for the future.

The Path Ahead

Given the vital importance of Positive Human Action and Positive Interaction for all people, all relationships and all life on our planet, we invest far too little time, money and energy on developing and implementing positive human development educational programs. We desperately need positive life enhancing resources and programs that can help all children, youth and adults live to their true potential and become the best and most positive human beings they can possibly be.

Very few schools and communities in the world are implementing meaningful and effective Positive Living Skills Education Initiatives. It is clear from our research that Positive Living Skills can help people of all ages become more focused learners, more fully connected performers, happier and more productive people, and more appreciative, respectful, relaxed human beings who are considerate and supportive of other people and the world around them (Amirault&Orlick, 1999; Gilbert &Orlick, 2002; Glynn, 2011; Hester &Orlick, 2006; Hjartarson, 2001;Klingenberg&Orlick, 2002; Koudys&Orlick, 2002; McMahon, Partridge, &Orlick, 2008; Orlick, 2014; Orlick& Partridge, 2008; Orlick, Zhou, &Partington, 1990; St. Denis &Orlick, 1996; Taylor &Orlick, 2004; Theberge, 2002). The challenges that we are currently facing in our schools, communities, countries, and greater world require that we develop and implement a global Positive Living Skills Educational Action plan. This Positive Global Action Plan is aimed at teaching all children and youth essential Positive Living Skills – including positive focusing skills for effective learning, positive focusing skills for quality performance, positive focusing skills for helping children and youth learn to be positive with themselves and others, and positive focusing skills to promote supportive and respectful living in school, at home, in their community, in their workplace, in their relationships, and beyond.

Our school systems, educational programs, educational and government leaders must give Positive Living Skills Education the attention it needs and deserves. The time has come to challenge ourselves, our school boards, our educational institutions, our leaders, our politicians, our decision makers, our media outlets, our teachers, our principals, our parents, our children, and our youth to implement and continue to improve positive educational initiatives that focus on teaching and nurturing essential skills for Positive Living, Positive Learning, Positive Interaction and Positive Performance. Let's implement the Positive Living Skills Program and continue to use, refine and improve our Positive Living Skills intiatives over the course of our lifetime and beyond.

We have an effective plan for teaching children and youth skills for positive living, which includes positive learning skills, positive performance skills, and skills for positive interaction and positive supportive communication with others. These skills include: positive focusing, positive refocusing, positive action plans, positive interaction plans, positive thinking, positive communication, positive ways of reducing and managing stress, positive ways to relax, positive distraction control, and fully connected focus training for enhanced learning, living, meaningful communication and improved performance.

People who are interested in creating a better and more compassionate world can begin to act on the Positive Living Skills Educational Initiative right now for the benefit of everyone. As long as we have the individual and collective will to make positive, life-enhancing changes, we can **do it**. Detailed information and specific program activities for school-based and home-based Positive Living Skills Education Program can be found in the following two books: (1) *Positive Living Skills: Joy and Focus for Everyone* (Orlick, 2011); and (2) *Happy Living Skills: Teachers and Parents Guide* (Orlick, 2014). There are also a series of educational audio CD tracks that were designed specifically to help teach children, youth, and adults Positive Living Skills and Positive Performance Skills (available on itunes – under Terry Orlick).

Our early research on the Positive Living Skills Program with elementary school children demonstrated that the PLS skills they were taught helped them to relax effectively, improve their stress control skills, focus on the positives in all situations, persevere through difficult situations, and experience more highlights or simple joys in their daily living. I have continued to refine and improve the Positive Living Skills program over the past 30 years and the content has been adapted to meet the needs of a variety of different age groups, from young children to teenagers, university students and adults (for more information on some of these studies see the following references: Gilbert &Orlick, 1996; Orlick, 1981a, 1981b, 1983, 2011; St. Denis &Orlick, 1996; Taylor &Orlick, 2004).

Positive Living Skills for Reducing Bullying Behaviors

In recent years, bullying has been identified as a significant and growing problem in many communities and schools throughout a variety of countries. Bullying and other negative behaviors have been acknowledged as having extremely detrimental effects on young peoples' physical and mental health (Blosnich&Bossarte, 2011). Bullying behaviors include negative physical acts, verbal abuse, social isolation and social exclusion (Durham District School Board, 2011). Cyber bullying has also been rapidly increasing in recent years and is having an outstandingly transparent negative impact (Sbarbaro&Enyeart Smith, 2011). The negative outcomes resulting from bullying behaviors include: elevated anxiety, depression, suicidal ideation, suicide, low self-esteem, feelings of loneliness, and social isolation (Kessel Schneider, O'Donnell, Stueve, & Coulter, 2012; Sbarbaro&Enyeart Smith, 2011; Whitted&Dupper, 2005), as well as lower academic achievement (Kessel Schneider et al., 2012).

Some studies have suggested that bullying behaviors may also be translated into displays of deviant behavior in adults such as alcoholism and criminal activity (Bowllan, 2011; Olweus, 1978; Whitted&Dupper, 2005). Clearly there is an urgent need to educate children in all parts of the world about positive living, so they can be educated and helped to grow into more positive and focused learners, better and more focused performers, less stressed and more relaxed individuals, more positive people, increasingly compassionate and caring human beings and productive contributors to a more humane world. This is the ultimate goal of the Positive Living Skills Global Initiative (Orlick, 2011).

A number of studies have highlighted the importance of introducing Positive Living Educational Programs to children and students while they are still young (Bowllan, 2011; Orlick, 1978, 1995, 2011; Sbarbaro&Enyeart Smith, 2011). Many children who learn to act in aggressive and negative ways early in life develop a variety of other problems including, but not limited to bullying, negativity and destructiveness towards themselves and others. If we can introduce effective and sustainable Positive Living Skills Programs to school children while they are still young, these children will have the opportunity learn and integrate empathy, relaxation, stress control, positive perspective, positive focus and positive self-control that will help them to recognize the value in themselves and the positives in others throughout their lives. Ongoing positive learning with a focus on positive personal growth can lead to healthier, happier and more joyful lives for virtually everyone (Olweus, 1978; Orlick, 1978, 2011, 2024; Orlick&Botterill, 1975).

Nurturing Positive Living Skills through Pro-active Positive Interventions

Implementing positive intervention programs to prevent or reduce negativity and enhance positive living has become an increasingly important goal to protect the health, mental well-being and security of all people. Bullying and other forms of highly negative and destructive behavior have gained major media attention because of their potential for having detrimental long-term effects on the physical and mental health of society. Bullying is a learned behavior. Infants are not born with the willful intent to hurt, degrade, harm or destroy other human beings. Therefore it is vitally important that we begin early childhood and youth positive education programs to prevent bullying or destructive behaviors before they are learned or adopted in the first place.

Blosnich and Bossarte (2011) found that bullying has become a behavior that negatively affects the lives of millions of people. There is an urgent need for immediate action to stem the rising tide of bullying and negativity in our schools, homes, neighborhoods and world at large. If our goal is to create and nurture a higher level of humanity (Orlick, 2002, 2011, 2014), the best time to begin a positive intervention option is when children are young so we can prevent negativity and bullying before it grows roots. By providing positive alternatives to negative ways of being at an early age, we are putting our children in a position to prevent negative actions or interactions before they occur. When we educate children about positive alternatives to negative ways of being, they have a much better chance of becoming positive, focused, successful, loving, caring and contributing human beings. As children learn how to focus in positive, considerate and fully connected ways, they become more compassionate human beings. In turn, this affects the quality of all children's lives. By introducing Positive Living Skills into our homes and schools, children will have a much better chance of becoming what they all have to potential to be - loving, caring, supportive, and productive human beings (Orlick, 2011, 2014).

We have spent many years developing a positive and practical educational program to help children and youth move forward in their lives in positive and life-enhancing ways. The Positive Living Skills Educational Program (PLSE) provides simple, positive educational activities to nurture positive human development; and it begins with children. We have also created and use a series of educational audio CD's to introduce various Positive Living Skills to children, youth and adults (Orlick, 2003a, 2003b, 2003c, 2003d, 2004, 2005a, 2005b, 2005c). The PLSE Program can be easily implemented right now in a range of school classroom contexts or in the homes of children and their families (Orlick, 2011, 2014).

The Positive Living Skills Educational Dream

The Positive Living Skills Program was designed to be relevant, enjoyable and life enhancing for all children, youth and adults. My dream is that we join together to teach Positive Living Skills to children and youth everywhere in the world so that their lives will have more harmony, less conflict, more positive focus, less negative focus, more connected focus, less disconnected focus, more joy, less unnecessary misery, more peace and harmony, less stress, more relaxation, less violence or conflict and more collaboration. My dream is that Positive waves of Positive Living will flow and extend throughout our homes, schools, playgrounds, relationships, communities, villages, neighborhoods, cities, and countries in all parts of our world. By teaching children to live, focus and interact in positive and compassionate ways, we can encourage a strong positive rippling effect across our immediate communities, countries, and eventually our world (Gilbert &Orlick, 2002, Orlick, 2014). This Positive Living path will lead us to more joyful and meaningful living and help all people learn to be happier, more relaxed, more fulfilled, more fully connected, more productive, more grounded and more joyful throughout the course of their lives. It will also empower children who have learned these Positive Living Skills to be in a wonderful position to teach others these skills and to be great role models for their own children when they become parents.

Children who are taught and encouraged to feel empathy and compassion for others at an early age have a much better chance of being compassionate contributors throughout the course of their lives. Positive Living Skills education helps children find good reasons to respect and support the positive qualities in others, but perhaps most important, it helps children to fully acknowledge, respect, and share the positive qualities within themselves. Children, youth and adults whose positive nature is nurtured and expanded upon have no reason to become bullies or negative people and will be in a wonderful positive to avoid becoming destructive towards themselves or others (Orlick, 2002, 2011, 2014).

Supporting the Goal of Positive Living

The Positive Living Skills program was designed to provide relevant educational activities for children and youth that lead to meaningful, positive real-world change in the lives of children and youth. The primary goal is to teach children how to live, learn, focus, perform, and interact with more joy, less stress, and a genuine sense of compassion for other people of all ages. Children have immense power and capacity to become positive agents of change in our world. We simply need to provide them with the tools, skills, and support to do so (Glynn, 2011; Orlick, 2002, 2011, 2014). I am a person who is very connected to nature and I often use the analogy of a flowing stream to illustrate the advantage of teaching positive living skills to children:

> "*A young child is like a pure and beautiful little stream of life. In positive unpolluted environments, little streams grow into powerful rivers, lakes or oceans and little children grow into strong, caring human beings who remain pure and clean. In negative or polluted environments, little streams and little people can become polluted, self-destructive and destructive towards others. We cannot wait for streams, rivers or people to become polluted or toxic and then attempt to clean them up. It is best to start when streams and children are small, pure, clean and free, and simply keep the doors open to help them continue to flow and grow in positive and live enhancing ways*" (Orlick, 2011, p. 9).

CONCLUSION

We have the capacity to change the world in positive and meaningful ways; and we have the capacity to do this right now! We have created and tested a Positive Human Development Educational Program that is capable of teaching Positive Living Skills to children and youth all over the world. We can instigate positive change quite easily by creating Positive Living Skills Leaders, and introducing the Positive Living Skills Educational Program to teachers throughout the world. These teachers and nurturers of Positive Living can then devote 20 to 25 minutes per day teaching the children in their classes Positive Living Skills. These positive teachings can then influence children to share their joy and positive knowledge, and encourage a ripple effect of positive living across the planet. We have the capacity and the simple educational resources to embark on this journey right now. All we need is the individual and collective will to DO IT!

REFERENCES

Amirault, K. & Orlick, T. (1999).Finding balance within excellence. *Journal of Excellence, 2,* 37-52.

Blosnich J. & Bossarte, R. (2011). Low-level violence in schools: Is there an association between school safety measures and peer victimization? *The Journal of School Health, 81*(2), 107-113. doi: 10.1111/j.1746-1561.2010.00567.x.

Bowllan, N. (2011). Implementation and evaluation of a comprehensive, school-wide bullying prevention program in an urban/suburban middle school.*Journal of School Health, 81*(4), 167–173.DOI:10.1111/j.1746-1561.2010.00576.x

Durham District School Board (2011).*Report bullying now!*Retrieved September 1, 2013, from http://www.ddsb.ca/Pages/newsitem.aspx?ItemID=48.

Gilbert, J. & Orlick, T. (1996). Evaluation of a life skills program with grade two children.*Elementary School Guidance and Counseling Journal, 31,* 139-151.

Gilbert, J. & Orlick, T. (2002).Teaching skills for stress control and positive thinking to elementary school children. *Journal of Excellence, 7,* 54-66.

Glynn, B. (2011). Stepping stones. *Journal of Excellence, 15,* 76-79.

Hester, K. & Orlick, T. (2006). The impact of a positive living skills training program on children with attention-deficit hyperactivity disorder. *Journal of Excellence, 11,* 4-31.

Hjartarson, F. (2001). Lessons learned: Mental training with young offenders and children at risk. *Journal of Excellence, 4,* 76-88.

Kessel Schneider, S., O'Donnell, L., Stueve, A., & Coulter, R. W. S. (2012). Cyberbullying, school bullying, and psychological distress: A regional census of high school students. *American Journal of Public Health, 102*(1), 171-177. doi:10.2105/AJPH.2011.300308

Klingenberg, M. & Orlick, T. (2002). Teaching positive living skills to a family with special needs.*Journal of Excellence, 7,* 5-35.

Koudys, J. & Orlick, T. (2002). Coping with cancer: Lessons from a pediatric cancer patient and his family. *Journal of Excellence, 7,* 36-53.

McMahon, S., Partridge, S. & Orlick, T. (2008). Positive living skills: Skating through adversity. *Journal of Excellence, 12,* 34-48.

Olweus, D. (1978). Aggression in the schools.*Aggressive Behavior, 5*(3), 309-311. doi:10.1002/1098-2337(1979)5:3<309:AID-AB2480050307>3.0.CO;2-S

Orlick, T. (1978). *The cooperative sports and games book.* New York, NY: Pantheon Publishers.

Orlick, T. (1981a). Cooperative play socialization among preschool children. *The Journal of Individual Psychology, 2*(1), 54-64.

Orlick, T. (1981b). Positive socialization via cooperative games. *Developmental Psychology, 17*(4), 426-29.

Orlick, T. (1983).Enhancing love and life mostly through play and games. *Journal of Humanistic Education and Development, 17*(4), 153-64.

Orlick, T. (1995). *Nice on my feelings: Nurturing the best in children and parents.* Carp, ON: Creative Bound Inc.

Orlick, T. (2002). Nurturing positive living skills for children: Feeding the heart and soul of humanity. *Journal of Excellence, 7,* 86–98.

Orlick, T. (2008). *In pursuit of excellence.* Champaign, IL: Human Kinetics Publishers.

Orlick, T. (2011). *Positive living skills: Joy and focus for everyone.* Renfrew, ON: General Store Publishing House.

Orlick, T. (2014). Happy living skills: Teachers and parents guide. *Zone of Excellence.* www.zoneofexcellence.ca.

Orlick, T. & Botterill, C. (1975). *Every kid can win: Nurturing the best in children and parents.* Chicago, IL: Nelson Hall Publishers.

Orlick, T. & Partridge, S. (2008). Positive living skills for teenagers: A youth intervention. *Journal of Excellence, 12*, 4-33.

Orlick, T., Zhou, Q. & Partington, J. (1990). Cooperation and conflict among Chinese and Canadian kindergarten children. *Canadian Journal of Behavioural Science. 22*(1), 20-25.

Sbarbaro, V. & Enyeart Smith, T. (2011). An exploratory study of bullying and cyberbullying behaviors among economically/educationally disadvantaged middle school students. *American Journal of Health Studies, 26*(3), 139-151.

St. Denis, M. & Orlick, T. (1996). Positive perspective intervention with fourth grade children. *Elementary School Guidance and Counseling Journal, 31*, 51-63.

Taylor, S. & Orlick, T. (2004). An analysis of a children's relaxation/stress control skills program in an alternative elementary school setting. *Journal of Excellence, 9*, 95-113.

Theberge, N. (2002). Mental skills training with children in a summer camp context. *Journal of Excellence, 7*, 76-85.

Whitted K. S. & Dupper, D. R. (2005). Best practices for preventing or reducing bullying in schools. *Children & Schools, 27*(3), 167-175.

Audio CDs

Orlick, T. (2003a). Audio CD 1. *Focusing for excellence: Relaxation and stress control activities.* Zone of Excellence.

Orlick, T. (2003b). Audio CD 2. *Focusing for excellence: Exercises for strengthening focus and performance.* Zone of Excellence.

Orlick, T. (2003c). Audio CD 2. *Focusing for excellence: Practicing in the zone.* Zone of Excellence.

Orlick, T. (2003d). Audio CD 2. *Focusing for excellence: Performing in the zone.* Zone of Excellence.

Orlick, T. (2004). Audio CD 1. *Spaghetti toes: Positive living skills for children.*

Orlick, T. (2005a). Audio CD 2. *Changing channels: Positive living skills for children.*

Orlick, T. (2005b). Audio CD 3. *Focusing through distractions: Positive living skills for tweens, teens and adults.*

Orlick, T. (2005c). Audio CD 4. *Relaxation and joyful living: Positive living skills for tweens, teens and adults.*

In: Positive Human Functioning ... Volume 2 ISBN: 978-1-62948-973-5
Editors: A. R. Gomes, R. Resende and A. Albuquerque © 2014 Nova Science Publishers, Inc.

Chapter 4

PROMOTING LIFE SKILLS IN CHILDREN AND YOUTH: APPLICATIONS TO SPORT CONTEXTS

Daniel Gould and Scott Westfall
Institute for the Study of Youth Sports, Michigan State University, Michigan, US

ABSTRACT

This chapter examines the research on using sport to promote life skills in children and youth and, based on this literature, derives implications for guiding practice. Specifically, the research and theory on factors associated with positive youth development across all out of school or after school activity program contexts is discussed. Next, the sport psychological research on promoting life skills through sport is reviewed. Example programs designed to promote life skills in children and youth through sport participation are discussed, as are theoretical explanations for how life skills are developed and influence young people. Finally, specific strategies and policies that can be used to promote life skills in children and youth through sport are examined. It is concluded that sport and physical activity contexts are wonderful places for promoting life skills. However, the development of life skills only occurs when these skills are systematically fostered and taught by caring, competent adults who use both direct and indirect strategies for doing so.

INTRODUCTION

Over the last two decades there has been a growing interest in examining how sport can be used to foster positive youth development and life skills in young people. This interest in sport and exercise psychology and related fields within Kinesiology has paralleled increased interest in the field of general psychology and youth development; fueled by the positive psychology movement which focuses on strength building versus deficit mending in people in general and youth in particular (Larson, 2000). While psychologists have only recently turned their attention to ways youth can build strengths, those in the sport world have long held firm beliefs about the role sport can play in youth development. For example, Barron Pierre de

Coubertin focused much of his rationale for the revitalization of the modern Olympic Games on the character-building virtues of sport (Kronspan, 2007). Moreover, youth sports programs around the world often emphasize the psychosocial benefits of sports participation for children and youth. For 40 years sport and physical activity researchers have also been studying ways psychosocial development occurs through participation in physical education and sport (Weiss, 2011). Hence, there is considerable interest in better understanding and using sport as a tool to enhance psychosocial attributes and life skills in young people.

While sport is widely believed by practitioners to be a major vehicle for development life skills, not all the evidence is supportive of their claims and some scholars suggest the claimed character and life skill benefits of sport are more myth than reality and/or are used by the industrial complex and those who have power in society to maintain their authority and influence. Coakley (2011), for example, has been highly critical of the character and life skills benefits of sport participation. Specifically, he has indicated that researchers studying the area have not been critical enough in examining the developmental effects on participants. Instead, they assume… "that, sport, unlike other activities, has fundamentally a positive and pure essence that transcends time and place so that positive changes befall individuals and groups that engage in or consume sport" (pp. 306-307)… He goes on to say "that collective claims of sport evangelists and their disciples are informed by neoliberal ideology focusing on personal development and success and discounting social issues and the need for progressive change at a collective or community level" (p. 308). However, Coakley (2011) is not the only critic. Hartman and Kwauk (2011) write that sport for development programs often focus on mainstream development practices conceived by program organizers who are not in touch with the communities these programs take place and for this reason ignore local knowledge and practices, as well as the needs and desires of the community and the sociocultural and political economic context. They often are designed to help the less fortunate better deal with their circumstances as opposed to helping empower these groups to solve the economic and social injustices that cause these problems in the first place. While these sociological concerns will not be the focus of this review they need to be recognized and examined to critically inform program development and implementation. They also remind us that we should not blindly assume that efforts to develop life skills through sport will have their intended positive effects just because we would like them to.

This chapter is designed to examine the research literature on using sport to promote life skills in children and youth and, based on this literature, implications for guiding practice are derived. This will be done by first summarizing the research and theory on factors associated with positive youth development across all out of school or after school activity program contexts. Next, sport psychological research on promoting life skills through sport will be reviewed for the purpose of critically examining the evidence for promoting life skills through sport. Third, example programs designed to promote life skills in children and youth through sport participation will be discussed. Fourth, theoretical explanations for how life skills are developed and influence young people are forwarded. Finally, specific strategies and policies that can be used to promote life skills in children and youth through sport will be examined.

Characteristics of Programs that Enhance Positive Youth Development

Researchers from a number of fields have been studying how participation in out-of-school and/or after school extracurricular activities such as music, drama, civic, religious groups or clubs influence young people. This interest arises from the popularity of these programs and from the fact that children and youth typically voluntarily engage in them and exhibit high levels of motivation relative to their involvement. They are also recognized as activities where young people have numerous opportunities to learn and perform in something deemed important to them and by society. Finally, these programs are thought to provide challenges and skill building opportunities for young people involved in them to meet (Larson, 2000).

Reviewing all the studies in this area is beyond the scope of this chapter. However, these studies typically involve surveying (e.g., Hansen & Larson, 2007) or interviewing young people involved in various activities and comparing them to young people engaged in different activities or not engaged at all (e.g., Dworkin, Larson, & Hansen, 2003). Some investigators have used qualitative methodologies, others quantitative, and still others mixed methods. Most studies involve cross-sectional assessments (e.g., Larson, Hansen, & Moneta, 2006) although a smaller number have involved longitudinal analyses (e.g., Eccles, Barber, Stone, & Hunt, 2003). Finally, a number of studies have evaluated the effectiveness of programs by treating them as interventions and making pre- and post-program measurements (e.g., Forneris, Danish, & Scott, 2007; O'Hearn & Gatz, 1999; 2002).

After reviewing the literature prior to 2002, the National Research Council and Institute for Medicine concluded that participating in these programs can have positive effects, especially when they were characterized by eight characteristics. These characteristics included: (1) a physically and psychologically safe environment; (2) a consistent and clear structure accompanied by adult supervision; (3) supportive relationships; (4) opportunities to belong; (5) positive social norms; (6) efficacy for mattering; (7) skill building opportunities; and (8) an integration of family, school and community efforts. Durlak, Weissberg, and Pachan (2010) conducted a meta-analysis of the literature focusing on the personal and social skills of children and youth who participated in out of school activities compared to controls who did not and found significant effects on variables such as school grades, reduced problem behaviors, positive social behaviors and school bonding. However, not all programs were effective – larger effects were found with programs that were sequenced, active, focused, and explicit. Mahoney, Vandell, Simpkins, and Zarrett (2009) also argue that effects are greatest for low-income children and youth. Hence, there is good evidence that participation in these programs can positively contribute to the development of young people, although effects are more likely to occur in programs of high quality and different activities may contribute more or less to differing outcomes with different groups of children.

Larson (2011) recently extended this area of research in an integrative review article where he examined the research on how youth develop various competencies in the real world by engaging in goal-oriented activities. Citing a series of recent longitudinal qualitative studies conducted by he and his colleagues (e.g., Larson & Brown, 2007; Larson & Walker, 2006; Wood, Larson, & Brown, 2009) a number of interesting conclusions and future directions were identified. Larson and Brown (2007), for example, propose that adolescents need to learn how to understand and manage emotions; and youth activity contexts, like participating in a theater production, are great places to do this. They also concluded that youth are agents of their own emotional development, emotional development occurs as a result of emotional hot episodes that naturally arise in activity settings, and youth come to understand and manage their emotions partly by drawing on the emotional environment that surrounds them and that this could be both constructive and unconstructive. In studying the development of responsibility in youth it was also noted that "…although program leaders often feel pressure to make activities fun, youth most likely experience gains in responsibility precisely from activities they complete that are challenging, onerous, and require self-discipline" (Wood et al., 2009, p. 306). Thus, developing life skills through activity participation may not always be fun and games. At times the experience will be a serious and emotionally taxing for the young people involved.

Turning to the development of the motivation needed to sustain goal-directed behavior Larson (2011) suggests that adolescents progress "from low motivation to personal connection to flow and sustained enjoyment" (p. 326). Youth, then, do not need to he highly motivated when they enter an activity setting. Larson (2011) also discusses cognitive development. Based on this team's research he suggests that cognitive development occurs by "doing" when youth actively experience the world by working on challenging projects and developing strategic thinking and flexible strategies for completing them.

Larson concludes his review of the literature by indicating that learning to navigate the complex and, often times, disorderly real world requires direct experiential learning and that positive youth development has many dimensions (e.g., interpersonal, ethical, civic). Six key points that cut across the different domains of development are also identified and should be considered when examining positive youth development associated with out-of-school activity participation. These include:

Point 1: Even as we learn more about the biological hardware of development, it is essential that we study the conscious software of youth development.

Point 2: We cannot understand adolescents' development without recognizing disorder any more than you can have physics without recognizing friction and entropy or biology without recognizing diversity and competition.

Point 3: Positive adolescent development requires knowledge and skills for navigating/dealing with/integrating/balancing heterogeneity and disorder.

Point 4: Adolescents are active "producers of their development."

Point 5: An individual's positive development is supported by processes across multiple bioecological (e.g., family, peers, school) systems.

Point 6: Research on development requires diverse methods to understand all the different parts of the elephant and how they are related (Larson, 2011, pp. 329-330).

RESEARCH ON PROMOTING LIFE SKILLS THROUGH SPORT

A number of researchers have been interested in understanding how psychosocial competencies and life skills are associated with participation in sport. Frist, a relatively small but highly committed group of developmental sport psychology researchers led by Maureen

Weiss and many of her students have been studying the development of psychosocial competencies, like perceived competence and moral development in children and youth (see Weiss, 2004, 2011, for overviews of this work) and while not often discussed as life skills are certainly related to the area. Over the last several decades, developmental psychologists have also looked at sport contexts as one of a number of out-of-school or after-school activities that may influence children and youth. An increasing number of researchers, then, have focused particular attention on the role involvement in sport plays on life skills development. Two major questions have been examined by these investigators: (1) what is the relationship between children and youth's life skills development and sport and physical activity involvement? And (2) what are factors that influence life skills development through sport and physical activity involvement? The research falling within each of these two general questions will be discussed below.

The Relationship between Life Skills Development and Sport and Physical Activity Involvement

Investigators have examined the relationship between sport and physical activity participation and life skills development, some using interviews and others using survey assessments. As part of a longitudinal study of the developmental influences of extracurricular activity involvement on youth, for example, Eccles and her colleagues (Eccles & Barber, 1999; Eccles et al, 2003) compared the influence of participating in school clubs, performing arts groups, church groups, academic clubs and team sports. Over 1.200 high school students were surveyed over a number of years and it was discovered that involvement in youth activities was related to positive educational orientations and lower rates of risky behaviors such as alcohol use. Sport participation, however, was found to be related to both positive and negative developmental experiences. On the positive side of the equation, team sports participation was associated with a number of desirable school outcomes (e.g., higher grade point, liking of school, college attendance). Those involved in sport were also found to engage in the risky behavior of drinking alcohol more often, as compared to other extracurricular activity involvement that was not found to be associated with any negative behaviors.

Dworkin et al. (2003) conducted a qualitative study to better understand the developmental outcomes youth reported from being involved in extracurricular activities. Focus groups were conducted with 55 adolescents who reported 6 major dimensions of development: exploration and identity work; development of initiative; emotional self-regulation; developing peer relationships and knowledge; teamwork and social skills; and adult networks and social capital. Thus, a wide range of learning was reported. Across the six domains the youth described themselves as active agents of the own development meaning that their development came from their own thoughts and actions. They also picked and choosed from what adults tried to teach them.

In follow-up study, Hansen, Larson, and Dworkin (2003) developed the Youth Experiences Scale, a measure of the developmental experiences young people have in extracurricular activities. In the initial study using the measure, a sample of 450 high school students completed the measure relative to three contexts in their lives: hanging out with friends, participating in structured youth activities (including sports), and participating in

Math or English class. When sports participation scores were examined relative to other youth activity contexts, higher rates of physical skills development, self-knowledge (e.g., learned what one is good at), and emotional regulation were found. However, negative peer interactions and inappropriate adult behavior (e.g., adults encouraged to do something they believed morally wrong) were more prevalent in the sport context. Sports involvement then was found to be associated with both positive and negative developmental experiences. It is interesting to note that in many of these studies sport is not only associated with the development of positive life skills but, at times, results in some negative consequences. This general finding is further verified in related areas of sport psychology research such as moral development (e.g., Shields & Bredemeir, 2007; Weiss, Smith, & Stuntz, 2008 for reviews) that shows participation in sport is often associated with an erosion of moral development in young people. Sport participants report learning bracketed morality where one develops a different view of what is consider moral inside versus outside of sport (e.g., fighting is more acceptable playing ice hockey but not in general life). Increased participation in sport is also associated with lower levels of moral development. At that same time, there is evidence that when the right social-emotional climate is created and/or good sporting behavior is intentionally taught moral behavior can be enhanced through sport participation.

In a study involving a large sample of young people (N = 2280), Larson, Hansen, and Moneta (2006) administered the Youth Experiences Scale-2, a self-report measure of developmental gains (e.g., identity development, emotional regulation) youth report from their non-school activity participation, and an activity participation questionnaire to high school students. Students participating in sports and arts activities were found to have higher YES-2 scores on the initiative subscale (e.g., experiences related to sustaining effort and setting goals). Sports participation was also related to higher self-reports of stress and athlete YES-2 scores were found to be more variable than the scores of the youth who reported being involved in other activities.

Carreres-Ponsoda, Carbonell, Cortell-Tormo, Fuster-Lloret, and Andreu-Cabrera, (2012) studied adolescents and compared the developmental benefits of participating in out-of-school sports, participation in other out-of-school activities, and participation in no out-of-school activities. In an interesting comparison they also examined youth who participated in sports plus other activities. It was found that youth who participated in the out-of-school sport programs had higher self-efficacy, personal and social responsibility and pro-social behaviors scores when compared to young people who participated in other activities or non activities. However, it was also found that those youth who participated in the sports plus activity group reported the highest levels of psychosocial skills while the youth who did not participate in any activity reported the lowest.

Several investigators have employed case study designs in an effort to better document and understand the process by which life skills are developed and the context surrounding those experiences. Holt, Tink, Mandigo, and Fox (2008), for example, studied one high school soccer team and its coach for the purpose of determining if and how life skills are developed. Field observations and in-depth interviews were conducted and it was revealed that coach embraced a philosophy of building relationships with the players. He also involved the players in decisions. The players reported that they developed teamwork and leadership, respect, and initiative through their experience. However, these skills were not found to be directly taught by the coach. Rather, the coach created opportunities for the players to use these life skills and then reinforced them when they occurred. When asked about the transferability of the life skills learned the players indicated that teamwork and leadership transferred to situations outside of soccer. The authors concluded that coaching life skills may be more about creating conditions where life skills can be player-generated, revealed and reinforced than about the direct teaching of these skills. They also indicated that adolescents with certain life skills are drawn to sport and through their sport participation further develop those skills that are then reinforced by their coaches.

Jones and Lavalee (2009) conducted a single case study of a 22 year-old female tennis player in an effort to determine how life skills were developed. Five formal and 30 hours of informal discussions took place. Interpretative analysis of the data revealed that the player perceived that her sports participation resulted in positive development. Furthermore, experiential learning was identified as the primary method life skills were developed, in that, training for and playing the game required the player to learn new life skills. It was also noted that dispositions (e.g., hard work, self-awareness) facilitated the learning of life skills and that the tennis experience reinforced her dispositions as well as taught her new life skills. The player also indicated that some life skills, like communication, transfer by building confidence across contexts. Thus, sport participation provided this athlete a context to both practice already developed life skills and dispositions and, at the same time, further develop them.

In addition to survey studies, investigators have also begun to design and test interventions for and/or evaluate the efficacy of promoting life skills in sport and physical activity settings. A series of studies in Greece, for example, have been conducted by Goudas and his colleagues (Goudas, Dermitzaki, Leondari, & Danish, 2006; Goudas & Giannoudis, 2008; Papacharisis, Goudas, Danish, & Theodorakis, 2005), who have tested either Danish's GOAL or SUPER life skill programs (Danish, 2002a; 2002b) in a series of experiments conducted in physical education and sport settings. Typical of these investigations was a two study project by Papacharisis and his colleagues (2005). Female youth volleyball (Study 1) and male soccer players (Study 2) were randomly assigned to an intervention or control condition with the intervention condition taking part in an 8 session abbreviated version of the SUPER Program that emphasized goal setting, problem solving and positive thinking. Results revealed that in both studies the intervention group improved and differed from the control group on sport specific skills, a knowledge test, and self-beliefs relative to goal setting, problem solving and positive thinking. Thus, the life skills intervention was shown to be effective. Similar results were found in their other studies conducted in physical education settings (Goudas et al., 2006; Goudas & Giannoudis, 2008).

In an experimental study using qualitative interviews, Brunelle, Danish, and Forneris (2007) examined the influence of a combined life skill program and community service on youth golfers. In the first part of the study, pre- versus post-intervention assessments showed that youth golfers receiving an intervention based on the SUPER program significantly increased their empathetic concern and social responsibility. Moreover, those in the intervention group who went on to do a community service project with the next six months (versus those who did not) further increased their pro-social values and community service orientations.

Weiss and her colleagues (Weiss, 2006; Weiss et al., 2013; www.firsttee.com) has also conduced an extensive evaluation of the First Tee life skills golf program. While the results of this project will be discussed later in this chapter, it is important to note that initial findings are encouraging as players were found to differ from comparison children on a variety of the life skills (e.g., honesty, responsibility, respect) contained in the program. Longitudinal data collected as part of the evaluation also showed that parents felt that a number of the life skills being taught in the program were transferring off the golf course and into other areas of the players' lives.

In summary, while more intervention and evaluation studies are needed, the research conducted to date shows that life skills interventions can be highly effective and are important in establishing causal relationships. Future studies should use better measures of life skills, more often take a longitudinal approach, and employ placebo control conditions. Hodge, Danish, and Martin (2012) also indicate that more emphasis should also be placed on assessing intervention fidelity and testing theoretical explanations for life skills development.

Factors Influencing Life Skills Development Through Sport and Physical Activity

A number of investigators have begun to study factors that may modify or influence the relationship between sport (and in some studies other activity) involvement and life skills development. For example, Hansen and Larson (2007) studied eleventh grade students using the YES measure and potential modifiers like dosage or degree of involvement, the ratio of the number of adults to youth in the program, taking on a lead role and motivation for involvement. Results revealed that having a lead role and a higher adult-to-youth ratio were related to a having a greater number of positive developmental experiences, as were greater levels of program dosage and the more youth indicated that they were motivated by enjoyment and the pursuit of future goals. Interestingly, activity type accounted for 25% of the variance in the number of developmental experiences reported while all of the modifying or what the investigators labeled amplifying factors accounted for 23% of the variance.

Several studies have been conducted to describe the characteristics and strategies used by high school coaches recognized for their ability to foster life skills in their athletes (Camire, Trudel, & Forneris, 2012; Gould, Collins, Lauer, & Chung, 2006, 2007; Gould, Voelker, & Griffes, 2013). Gould and his colleagues (2006, 2007) interviewed 10 high school football coaches, who were recognized for their influence on the personal development of their players. Results revealed that the coaches used a variety of life skills coaching strategies. These included both direct (e.g., discussing important values with their players) and indirect strategies (e.g., creating an environment that emphasizes their key core values). The coaches also took an integrated approach to their life skills development efforts as they did not separate life skills coaching from their general coaching duties. Based on their findings, Gould and his colleagues also derived a four-stage model explaining how these coaches fostered life skills. First, these coaches espoused coaching philosophies that placed considerable importance on life skills development. Second, they fostered strong coach-athlete relationships. Third, they utilized specific life skills strategies that were in line with their core values. Finally, the coaches considered the specific context in which their athletes lived and adapted their life skills coaching efforts accordingly.

Camire and his colleagues (2012) extended the research of Gould and his colleagues when they interviewed 9 experienced coaches and 16 of their student-athletes. The results were consistent with the model forwarded by Gould et al. (2006), in that the coaches had philosophies that featured life skills development at their core. They also formed strong relationships with their athletes and had specific strategies for teaching the life skills they valued. In addition to supporting the Gould et al. life skills coaching model, Camire et al. (2012) found that the coaches believed their student athletes could transfer the life skills they learned through sport and reported taking steps to educate their athletes about transferring life skills.

Finally, in a study examining coaches who were know for fostering the particular life skill of leadership in their youth captains, Gould, Voelker, and Griffes. (2013) interviewed 10 experienced high school coaches. Findings showed that these coaches were proactive about intentionally teaching their student-athletes about being a leader in general and captain in particular. Strategies included teaching them how to communicate effectively, holding regular coach-captain meetings, providing examples of good leaders, giving the captains real responsibilities and conducting formal leader training sessions outside of practice. They also recommended that coaches who wanted to develop their captains develop strong leadership philosophies, be proactive in training captains and empower their captains by giving them autonomy in carry out their leadership responsibilities.

Gould and Carson (2010, 2011) also conducted several quantitative studies focusing on how coaches influence the development of life skills. Specifically, their studies were designed to better understand how perceived coaching attitudes and behaviors (e.g., the degree coaches focused on and taught mental preparation, goal setting, competition strategies, physical training and planning, coach-athlete rapport) were associated with life skills development as assessed by the YES-2. High school athletes were used in both studies and completed the YES-2 and a measure of the perceived frequency of various coaching behaviors. Results revealed that young athletes who reported higher levels of the perceived coaching behaviors like goal setting, teaching competition strategies, talking about how sport lessons related to life and building positive rapport with their athletes also reported greater levels of life skills like emotional regulation, cognitive skills, feedback, pro social norms and community linkages. Across the two studies, then, the results clearly showed that perceived coaching behaviors were significantly related to the development of life skills in scholastic athletes. The authors also argued that it makes intuitive sense that coaches who teach their players more about goal setting, mental preparation strategies, and emphasize hard work would have student-athletes who reported more learning related goal setting, effort and emotional regulation. Similarly, coaches who emphasize life skills development (e.g., model good sportsmanship, talk to their athletes about how sport lessons relate to life) would have players who do not report inappropriate adult experiences. Finally, having a strong positive rapport with one's athletes was an important and consistent predictor of reported life skills.

In a third study in this line of research, Gould, Flett, and Lauer (2012) recently measured the developmental outcomes underserved youth reported from their sports participation. The YES-2 was given to 239 urban youth baseball and softball participants, as well as measures of the sports climate with specific emphasis placed on assessing the motivation and caring aspects of the climate created, as well as measures of the importance their coaches placed on life skills. Results revealed that significant relationships were found between YES-2 scales and subscales and the motivation and caring climate predictor variables. Specifically the more coaches were perceived to have created a caring, mastery-oriented climate, the more likely athletes reported positive life skills development (e.g., teamwork and social skills, initiative). Ego oriented climates were found to be related to negative experiences like inappropriate adult relationships and social exclusion. A number of the previous findings of Gould and Carson (2010, 2011) were also supported.

Recently, Bruner, Hall, and Côté (2011) examined the relationship between sport type (basketball versus middle-distance running) and task interdependence (where it is perceived that an individual's performance is dependent on others) and outcome interdependence (where it is perceived that the benefits one derives from participation is dependent on others performance) on YES-2 assessments of 212 athletes, ages 14-17. While some sport type differences in YES-2 subscale scores were reported (e.g., basketball players reported higher teamwork and social skills) when sport type was controlled perceptions of outcome interdependence significantly predicted a number of developmental experiences. This led the authors to conclude that while different sports may provide different learning experiences for youth, their developmental experiences may be more strongly related to how the people in sport interact with one another (their task outcome interdependence).

Finally, Strachan, Côté, and Deakin (2009) conducted a study to determine if youth who specialize in sport versus those who do not differ in the developmental benefits that are derived. Young athletes (34 samplers and 40 specializers) were administered the Youth Experiences Scale-2 and comparisons were made between the groups. Findings revealed that the groups did not differ in their sources of enjoyment. However, the samplers reported more experiences on the linkages to the community and integration of the family subscales while specializers reported more experiences with diverse peer groups and being more burned out. The authors concluded that because the sample size was small, results need to be interpreted with some caution. Moreover, while some differences existed between the samplers and specializers the groups were more similar than different in the developmental benefits they derive from sport.

In summary, the research examining factors that influence the development of life skills in young athletes shows that the perceived actions and values of coaches are the factor that most consistently influenced the development of life skills across multiple studies. Specifically, coaches who have a greater influence on life skill development are characterized by having philosophies that place primary importance on life skills development, emphasize sportsmanship to a greater degree, were proactive about teaching life skills, were able to form strong relationships with their players, focused more on teaching skills like goal setting, mental preparation, and competitive strategies, and discussed the importance of transferring life skills to other settings more often. They also placed a stronger emphasis on creating a caring and task orientated motivational climate and emphasized physical training. Other factors that have been identified as predictors of life skill development include players taking a lead role, higher adult to youth ratios, higher program dosages and athletes perceiving greater task interdependence. These factors, however, need to be further verified in future studies.

THEORETICAL EXPLANATIONS FOR LIFE SKILLS DEVELOPMENT

While there has been considerable interest in studying life skills, theory development efforts have lagged behind. After reviewing the literature, Gould and Carson (2008) complied a heuristic model explaining how life skills influence athletes. Specifically, they argue that athletes do not enter sport without already developed or partially developed life skills and psychosocial attributes and these skills and attributes influence the life skills development through sport process. Thus, they suggest that the young person's pre-existing internal and external assets influence his or her life skills development. They further argue the life skills are developed through the sport experience and this experience is influenced by coach characteristics, as well as the coaches' direct and indirect life skills coaching strategies that can lead to both positive and negative physical, mental and psychosocial outcomes. However, they also propose a number of explanations for why life skills develop. These include environmental explanations like an enhanced sense of belonging, peer influences or positive social norms, as well as the utility of the life skill itself (e.g., goal setting helps the athlete achieve better performance). Finally, Gould and Carson include a component of the model that focuses on the transferability of the psychosocial attributes and life skills to other settings, outlining factors which are likely to influence this process (e.g., confidence in one's ability to perform the life skill, a belief that the life skill is valuable). The Gould and Carson model, then, summarizes much of the current research on life skills development. However, they did not make specific predictions to be tested.

Recently Hodge et al. (in press) have developed a conceptual model to explain life skills interventions. The model builds from on an earlier explanation for lifespan development interventions developed by Danish and D'Augelli (1983) and self-determination theory (Deci & Ryan, 2002, 2008). It is contented that when the autonomy, competence, and relatedness basic needs are met and a needs-supportive motivational climate exists athletes experience positive psychological development, the outcome objective for most life skills programs. They further contend that the more one internalizes the basic needs of autonomy, competence, and relatedness the more generalized life skills will be developed and transferred to other contexts like school or to family settings.

While the Gould and Carson (2008) and Hodge et al. (in press) models provide a good beginning to providing explanations for life skills development, they are only a start. More theory development work is needed.

Sample Programs Designed to Promote Life Skills in Children and Youth Through Sport

There are many sport programs that focus on developing psychosocial competencies and life skills in children and youth. Some are large national and international programs, like golf's The First Tee, that have standardized curriculums, are delivered at numerous sites around the world, and influence thousands of young people. Others like, Project Effort at the University of North Carolina Greensboro involve a small number of youth in an after school physical activity club with no standardized curriculum or national backing. It would be beyond the scope of this chapter to review all these programs. However, in this section several programs will be briefly described to provide a sense of their purposes, the content delivered, and how they are organized and implemented. These programs were also selected because they have all been subject to some type of program evaluation, something that happens to infrequently in the life skills through sport research.

Detroit Police Athletic League

The Detroit Police Athletic League (DPAL) is a non-profit sports program in Detroit, Michigan, with the primary goal of character development. It serves approximately 10.000, mostly underserved youth. DPAL also trains 1,000 adults who serve as coaches and managers in its many sports programs. The primary goal of DPAL is to transform youth through sport participation by: promoting positive character development in young people who participate; promoting the development of positive life skills, physical fitness, and healthy lifestyles; and helping young people grow into healthy adults. DPAL programming is measured against five points of excellence: fair opportunities for boys and girls; positive family environment; safe and clean fields and facilities; superior sportsmanship; and, consistent attention to detail. DPAL achieves its objectives by running traditional sports programs. However, its coaches are trained in principles of positive youth development with this training focusing on equipping coaches with the knowledge and tools needed to develop five attributes in program participants: (1) a sense of purpose and positive view of the future; (2) responsibility; (3) integrity; (4) perseverance; and (5) compassion. DPAL also has paid Detroit Police officers, who have received special training, serve as Youth Development Officers YDO). YDOs' run special mentoring programs for the young athletes and coaches, and conduct a captains circle program where youth captains received leadership training.

DPAL has been collecting evaluation data to assess if it is achieving its goals (Bean, Whitley, & Gould, in press; Flett, Gould, Griffes, & Lauer, 2012; in press; Flett, Gould, & Lauer, 2012; Gould et al., 2012; Whitley, Bean, & Gould, 2011). This data has generally been supportive, although an effort has also been made to identify aspects of the program that are ineffective and need to be addressed (see Flett, Gould, Griffes, & Lauer, in press).

Goal and Sports United to Promote Education and Recreation

The Going for the Goal Program (GOAL) is one of the oldest life skills training programs and has been used both in sport and other contexts. It was developed by Steve Danish, a pioneer in the life skills through sport movement and Director of the Virginia Commonwealth University Life Skills Center. The program has received a number of national honors, including the National Mental Health Association Lela Rowland Prevention Award. The GOAL program is a 10-hour program that focuses on enhancing participants' sense of confidence and personal control. A forerunner of the positive psychology movement the GOAL program helps youth know "what to say yes to" versus "just saying no." A number of skills are taught in the program, typically by older peers. Some of these include: (1) the identification of positive life goals; (2) a process versus outcome focus to goal setting; (3) problem-solving; (4) the identification of behaviors that will interfere with goal achievement; (5) the identification of behaviors that can facilitate goal achievement; (6) understanding and seeking out social support; and (7) the transference of the life skills learned. Materials have been developed for those who implement the goal program and a formal process for doing so is in place.

A related program was also developed by Danish and the Life Skills Center staff; the Sports United to Promote Education and Recreation (SUPER) program. This character- based program is taught through a sports clinic where young athletes receive 18 different modules.

Learning activities are related to: the physical skills related to a specific sport; life skills (related to sports); and playing the sport. The program is designed to teach the athletes mental skills like goal setting, problem solving, and how to use social support that can be used in sport and life. Several of the SUPER modules are based on the GOAL program.

Several studies have been conducted to test the efficacy of the GOAL and SUPER programs both in sport (Brunelle et al., 2007; Goudas et al., 2006; Goudas & Giannoudis, 2008; Papacharisis et al., 2005) and in general (O'Hearn & Gatz, 1999, 2002). Papacharisis et al. (2005), for example in a previously discussed study, found that a shortened version of the SUPER program was effective in increasing life skills knowledge, greater problem solving, constructive thinking about goal setting (all skills taught) and performance when intervention group participants were compared to controls.

Teaching Personal and Social Responsibility Programs

There are a large number of sport and physical activity-based programs (see Hellison & Cutforth, 1997 for an example) that have adopted Hellison's (2011) teaching personal and social responsibility (TSPR) model for developing youth. Hellison's model focuses on helping youth learn personal and social responsibility in stages by: (1) achieving self-control and respect for others; (2) giving good effort and participating; (3) becoming self-directed; and (4) helping others. This process is facilitated by instructors who use strategies like providing relational time, awareness talks, group meetings, and reflection time. In the book, *Teaching responsibility through physical activity* Hellison (2011) discusses program assumptions, core values, levels of responsibility, and program leadership.

It is important to note that while TPSR is a widely used model to guide life skills programs there is no national curriculum or standardized format for the program. Instead, local implementers individualize the model to fit their own needs. TSPR programs also tend to be small, single sight operations and have typically involved physical education classes or informal noncompetitive sport and physical activity clubs. A number of, mostly qualitative research studies have been conducted on programs using the model and shown that it to be generally effective (see Hellison & Cutforth, 2002). A quantitative scale has also been developed to measure TPSR with encouraging initial results (Li, Wright, Rukavina, & Pickerning, 2008; Watson, Newton, & Kim, 2003).

Play It Smart

The Play It Smart Program was developed by the National Football Foundation for the purpose of meeting the academic and life skill needs of disadvantaged high school football players. Based on the life skills development model (Danish, Petitpas, & Hale, 1993), program participants are taught to identify transferable skills from sport. They then learn how to apply these skills to their academic preparation. Individual and group goal setting is applied. The main delivers of the program are academic coaches who work 20 hours a week coordinating and delivering the program. In addition to supporting the athletes academically, the academic-coaches conduct team-building activities (e.g., ropes courses, community service projects) to build a sense of community and foster constructive and positive group norm.

Initial data collected as part of the Play It Smart two-year pilot program showed that grade point average and graduate rates of program participants increased over controls (Petitpas, Van Raalte, Cornelius, & Presbrey, 2004). The participants were also more likely to attend college and engaged in a high number of community service hours.

The First Tee

One of, if not the largest life skills through sport development programs is the First Tee. The program is designed to introduce youth "...to the game of golf and its inherent values" and is designed to "impact the lives of young people by providing educational programs that build character, instill life-enhancing values and provide healthy choices through the game of golf" (see: www. FirstTee.com). Built around the nine core values of honesty, integrity, sportsmanship, respect, confidence, responsibility, persistence, courtesy, and judgment the program is implemented in a variety of educational and after school programs around the world. Through a well-thought out three level program, participants learn from trained instructors how to manage emotions, resolve conflict, set goals, introduce ones self, and communicate with others.

The First Tee program has also undergone a rigorous mixed method evaluation conducted by noted developmental sport psychologists, Maureen Weiss and her team of researchers from the University of Minnesota. While publications are only now coming out on the project, these initial scientific findings (Weiss, 2011; Weiss, Stuntz, Bhalla et al., 2013) and those reported on The First Tee website are very encouraging. In particular it has been found that after three years in the program 73% of the participants reported higher confidence in their ability to do well academically while 82% felt confident in their social skills. Participants also indicated that they demonstrated honesty (62%), acted personally and socially responsible (61%), and were respectful towards themselves and others (59%). When compared to non First Tee controls, First Tee players scored significantly higher on life skills like goal-setting, initiative, and managing emotions. They also scored higher on demonstrating positive character traits and measures of life skills transfer.

Strategies and Policies for Promoting Life Skills in Children and Youth Through Sport

The research examining the development of psychosocial attributes and life skills through sport has a number of implications for those interested in promoting positive development in children and youth. These include: (1) creating a conducive environment for life skills development; (2) emphasizing the intentional teaching of life skills; (3) selecting coaches with the right philosophy and coaching competencies; (4) fostering strong coach-athlete relationships; (5) coordinating sport-based life skills development efforts with other significant others and agencies in the young athlete's community; (6) teaching for transfer; (7) using logic models to design and understand life skills interventions and programming;

and (8) evaluating the efficacy of life skill development efforts. Each of these general strategies will be discussed below.

Creating a Conducive Environment

Life skills and psychosocial competencies are most likely to be developed in young athletes when they participate in environments that are conducive to the development of these skills and dispositions. For example, research from the general field of youth development suggests that positive development is most likely to occur when physically and psychologically safe environments are provided, when programs have a consistent and clear structure accompanied by adult supervision, when supportive relationships occur, when children and youth have opportunities to belong, when positive social norms exist, children experience an efficacy for mattering, there are skill building opportunities, and when programs are integrated with other external assets like the family, school and community efforts (National Research Council and Institute for Medicine, 2002). The more these conditions are created the more successful programs will likely be in promoting life skills in children and youth.

Using the general youth development literature as a base, Petitpas et al. (2005) have emphasized that it is especially important for those creating sport and physical activity-based life skills programs to consider the type of sport context they will be working in. For example, programs focused on teaching personal and social responsibility in an informal out of school physical activity club setting are able to organize, design and even modify the games and sports being taught for the specific purpose of teaching life skills. However, those wanting to teach life skills within a high school athletics context have less flexibility in modifying rules, the game or the structure of competition. These programs also have multiple goals and objectives (e.g., enhanced fitness, winning, the acquisition of sports skills) beyond the development of life skills that must be considered. Thus, while the research has shown that life skills can be fostered in young people in both contexts, practitioners must consider how the program context will influence their life skills development efforts and plan programs accordingly.

One environmental factor that has been repeatedly linked to enhanced life skills development in children and youth participating in sport and physical activity contexts is the motivational climate created by the teacher or coach (Duda, & Balaguer, 2007; Smith, Smoll, & Cummings, 2007). The more the climate is task-oriented, provides autonomy of choice, and enhances enjoyment and positive adult-peer relationships, the more likely life skills will be developed. Over emphasizing winning, employing authoritarian and harsh coaching practices, and engaging in constant social comparison is not conducive to life skill development. It is especially important to provide youth agency by giving them developmentally appropriate levels of autonomy and choice and by minimizing adult control. Of course, given some of the inherent physical dangers in sport (e.g., balls being thrown, difficult skills being learned) this needs to be done in a way where adult leaders can meet their legal and ethical responsibility of providing a physically and safe participation environment.

Emphasizing the Intentional Teaching of Life Skills

While some research suggests that young people learn life skills on their own, via an implicit process arising from the experience of playing sport (Holt, Tamminen, Tink & Black, 2009; Jones & Lavalle, 2009), most experts in the field contend that optimal development results when coaches, parents and administrators are very intentional in their life skills teaching efforts. Weiss (2011) summed this up best when she said that that children and youth best develop psychosocial and behavioral competencies when an "appropriate structure and an intentional curriculum that provides clear and consistent rules and expectations, adult supervision, guidance and age appropriate monitoring and a climate that allows for physical and psychological safety" is provided (p. 59). Studies of coaches who are effective at teaching life skills, for example, show that these individuals identify specific life skills they intend to foster in their athletes while at the same time implementing specific strategies for fostering these skills (Camire et al., 2012; Gould et al., 2007). Less effective or experienced coaches often report lofty life skills objectives but are unable to identify specific strategies for fostering these goals (McCallister, Blinde, & Weiss, 2000) or do not demonstrate the life skills themselves (Flett et al., in press). Life skills based physical education and activity interventions shown to be effective also focus on specific life skills implementing intentional strategies for achieving them (e.g., Wright & Burton, 2008).

Selecting Coaches with the "Right" Philosophy and Competencies

If life skills are to be fostered in young people it is especially important to select teachers and coaches who are guided by the "right" philosophy. They must place primary importance on developing life skills (Camire et al., 2012; Collins, Gould, Lauer, & Chung, 2009) and be committed to creating environments to teach these skills and values. These individuals must also posses the skills and competencies that allow them to foster strong coach-athlete relationships, utilize direct and indirect life skills teaching strategies, and teach for transfer. Finally, they must be open to engaging in coaching education efforts to increase their life skills coaching competencies.

It is encouraging the recent research by MacDonald, Côté, and Deakin (2010) has shown that coach training is associated with higher rates of personal and social competencies in young athletes. In particular, informal coach training in the form of discussing positive youth development at coaching meetings and through coach to coach mentoring was related to personal and social skills development.

Building Relationships

One of the most consistent findings in life skills development through sport research is that life skills are most likely to be developed in young people when they perceive a strong coach-athlete relationship (Camire et al., 2012; Gould & Carson, 2010, 2011; Gould et al., 2012). Moreover, this can be done by striving to understand and learn about one's athletes, engaging in team building activities, having athletes keep journals and sharing their responses with their coach, and gaining the athletes respect by being a competent coach (Camire,

Forneris, Trudel, & Bernard, 2011). Young athletes also want their coaches to interact with them in a positive upbeat fashion (Whitley, Bean, & Gould, 2011).

Finally, part of fostering a positive coach-athlete relationship is to creating a caring climate (Fry & Gano-Overway, 2010; Fry, Guivernau, Kim, Newton, Gano-Overway, & Magyar, 2011). This can be accomplished by making sure one connects with "each" young athlete in a caring and supportive manner, setting clear expectations relative to the team climate for all to hear, and facilitating positive relationships between athletes and parents of young athletes (Fry, 2010). Moreover, while much of the literature focuses on a strength based approach to youth development in sport, this does not mean problems or potential problems are ignored. Waldron (2012), for instance, has stressed how important it is for coaches to be proactive in efforts to prevent negative behaviors such as hazing. In particular, she recommends that coaches hold workshops for their athletes where hazing is clearly defined and discussed, team norms are established to distinguish hazing from appropriate team rituals, and athletes be taught steps for recognizing, reporting and taking steps to prevent and/or stop hazing practices in sport.

Coordinating Life Skills Development Efforts with other Individuals and Agencies in Athletes Communities

Young athletes do not live in a sport vacuum. They exist within a complex social system and are influenced by many individuals (parents, peers, teachers) and agencies (family, school, community). It is not surprising, then, that the more external assets a child experiences the more likely positive development takes place (Benson & Saito, 2000). For this reason, coaches and teachers desiring to help their students and athletes develop life skills should work to coordinate efforts with other significant others and agencies that the child is influenced by. This might involve encouraging young athletes to participate in other activities and asking them how things are going with their involvement, when possible learn what is being emphasized in those activities, and meeting individuals who run those activities. Forneris, Camire, and Trudel (2012) have also emphasized the importance of school-based coaches understanding the mission of their school and their athletic program and making efforts to align their life skills coaching efforts to large school goals. Finally, efforts should be made to inform parents of one's life skills coaching objectives and solicit their help in providing feedback about athlete development in these areas, as well as providing any information about the child that will help coaches reach their life skills development goals for their young athletes.

Teaching for Transfer

Gould and Carson (2008) have argued that for psychosocial competencies or skills to truly qualify as a life skill the young person must transfer these skills from the physical activity or sport context to other life settings such as school or to their part time job. Recent research has shown that young athletes report that they transfer some of the lessons learned in sport to other aspects of their life (Camire et al., 2009, 2012; Holt et al., 2009; Jones & Lavalle, 2009). While athletes may do this on their own accord, transfer is much more likely to occur if teachers and coaches intentionally teach for transfer. It is encouraging that it has been recently shown that model high school coaches report having specific strategies for teaching student-athletes about the transferability of the life skills they learn (Camire et al., 2012). Research by Weiss (2006) with First Tee golf program participants, parents and coaches has also found strong evidence of life skills taught in the program transferring from the golf course to home, in school, in various social situations and at the workplace. Strong evidence for 'meet and greet' skills, strategies for managing negative thoughts, emotions and behaviors, and a greater appreciation and understanding of diversity were found. This was not surprising as these behaviors were intentionally taught in the program.

However, transfer is not automatic. Several studies have found that transfer tends to be variable (e.g., Martinek, Schilling, & Johnson, 2001). For example, Martinek and his associates (2001) in looking at an after school physical activity based life skills program found that some participant behaviors were more successfully transferred to the school setting than others. Moreover, Camire et al. (2012), while reporting that the coaches and student athletes they interviewed felt that the life skills learned in sport can transfer to other settings, variations were reported depending on the student's characteristics and maturity.

Relative to strategies for teaching for life skills transfer, Danish, Taylor, and Fazio (2003) in designing various physical activity and sport-based life skills programs have facilitated the development and transfer by employing several strategies. First, within the program they ensure the instructors discuss how the life skills being taught link to sport performance. They also provide examples and demonstrations of how these skills are practiced and cultivated both inside and outside of sport. Third, opportunities for athletes to practice these skills within the sport setting are created. Fourth, they help the young athletes develop and implement a plan for utilizing the skills learned outside of sport. Finally, time is spent debriefing with the young athletes where successes and failures of using the various life skills in both sport and other life contexts are discussed.

Gass (1985) writing in the adventure-based learning area has also identified conditions needed to transfer life skills. These include having the participant learn the specific skills and qualities being focused on; having the individual recognize that he or she posses those skills and qualities; providing opportunities to test the skills in a safe setting; and, lastly, making on effort to transfer their skills.

Using Logic Models to Guide Interventions

An excellent way for practitioners, especially those working at the programmatic level where multiple individuals will be delivering a life skills program to different teams or groups of youth, is to employ a logic model (Wells & Arthur-Banning, 2008). Logic models are used in a variety of fields and involve visually displaying how one's program works by having the provider identify resources or inputs (e.g., qualified volunteers to coach), activities (e.g., coach training program), outputs (e.g., passing coach certification test), outcomes (e.g., increase in positive coach-athlete relationship) and impacts (increase in athlete initiative or emotional control) (W. K. Kellogg Foundation, 2004). By developing a well thought out logic model practitioners find that the rationale behind their program is clarified, critical aspects of the program are determined, organizers better understand how the program works, and evaluation of the program is facilitated.

Keeping Score through Program Evaluation

Petitpas and his colleagues (2005) have stressed the importance of evaluating sport and physical activity based efforts to foster psychosocial and life skills development in young athletes. This is especially important for large program efforts, typically funded by Foundations or government agencies, as in today's world organizations are expected to have evidence to back up any life skills development claims. We recommend using both qualitative and quantitative methods as it allows us to understand the scale and scope of effects while at the same time helping explain why effects occur and how individuals may idiosyncratically respond to life skills development efforts.

Evaluation should not be limited to large programmatic efforts, however. Individual coaches and teachers should be making efforts to evaluate their efforts, albeit in a less formal matter. This might include interviewing athletes who age out or graduate from programs for the purpose of obtaining feedback about life skills training activities. Similarly, coaches might make efforts to track how their athletes are doing at school by checking attendance, academic progress and any disciplinary actions. Talking to teachers and parents and learning whether the young athletes are exhibiting any of the skills taught are another way to evaluate whether life skills are being developed.

WHERE TO FROM HERE: THE FUTURE OF PROMOTING LIFE SKILLS THROUGH SPORT

This review leads to a number of recommendations for promoting life skills through sport. First, the literature shows that there is a clear link between sport participation, especially when life skills are given central importance and intentionally fostered, and participation in youth sports. Thus, life skills can and should be developed in children and youth through youth sports participation.

Our review has also shown that intervention studies using experimental designs provide initial evidence that this relationship is causal, albeit most likely reciprocal, in that, young people enter sport and physical activity programs with certain dispositions, values and life skills in hand that influence the development of life skills from that program at the same time having those dispositions, values and skills reinforced and modified from the sport experience itself. New life skills and orientations can also be developed through participation.

Third, coaches and other physical activity providers who appear to be more effective at promoting life skills in children and youth have philosophies that place prime importance on life skills, values, and related dispositions as key objectives of sports participation. While some evidence shows that life skills might be developed through interaction with peers and the child's own action, they are much more likely to occur if they are intentionally taught and fostered.

The evidence is also showing that coaches' ability to develop positive rapport, caring, and trusting relationships with the young people is essential for developing life skills. The adage, that young people engaged in sport "don't care what you know, until they know what you care" certainly applies when one is interested in promoting and fostering life skills through sport in young people.

Task oriented, supportive climates have also been linked to life skills development, as has been the need for autonomy supporting environments. Authoritarian, outcome focused ego oriented climates do not make conducive settings of life skills development.

It should also be recognized that life skills are promoted in young people through both direct and indirect teaching and coaching actions of adult leaders. This occurs indirectly through, the context and motivational climate created in the program, as conditions are created that allow children and youth to have experiences that more likely lead to life skills development. Direct coaching actions like specifically discussing life skills with young people, teaching specific life skills, and reinforcing them when they occur are all examples of direct strategies for teaching and promoting life skills in young people and should be emphasized.

The latest thinking and research is also showing that if dispositions, values and skills are to be life skills and influence child in other life contexts, then practitioners must teach for transfer. For example, they must talk about how life skills can apply outside of the sport context and encourage and help athletes engage in efforts to transfer these skills and values.

Coordinating life skills development efforts with other significant others and agencies in young athletes communities greatly increases the likelihood that these skills will be effectively developed. The old adage, "it takes a village to raise a child" applies to fostering and promoting life skills in young people.

Finally, practitioners are encouraged to develop logic models to help crystalize their goals and help orient their thinking and actions about how there program will specifically impact the development of life skills. They should also make efforts to practically evaluate if they are reaching their goals as developing life skills is a complex process and not every strategy will lead to the intended outcome.

It is our opinion, then, that sport and physical activity contexts are wonderful places for promoting life skills in children and youth. Therefore, more needs to be done to make sure this occurs. We must guard against blinding assuming that because sport was good personally for many of us relative to the learning of life skills, it will be good for all children and youth who participate. Sport does not teach life skills. It is those of us who organize, coach and carry out sport that create the conditions for doing so. We must do more to intentionally and systematically make this happen!

REFERENCES

Bean, E., Whitley, M., & Gould, D. (in press). Athlete impressions of a character-based sports program for underserved youth. *Journal of Sport Behavior, 37*(1).

Benson, P., & Saito, R. (2000). The scientific foundation of youth development. In N. Jaffe & J. Marquis (Eds.). *Youth development: Issues, challenges and directions* (pp. 126-147). Philadelphia, PA: Public/Private Ventures.

Brunelle, J., Danish, S. J., & Forneris, T. (2007). The impact of a sport-based life skill program on adolescent prosocial values. *Applied Developmental Science, 11*, 43-55.

Bruner, M. W., Hall, J., & Côté, J. (2011). Influence of sport type and interdependence on the developmental experiences of youth male athletes. *European Journal of Sport Science, 11*(2), 131-142.

Camire, M., Forneris, T., Trudel, P., & Bernard, D. (2011). Strategies for helping coaches facilitate positive youth development through sport. *Journal of Sport Psychology in Action, 2*(2), 92-99.

Camire, M., Trudel, P., & Forneris, T. (2009). High school athletes' perspectives on support, communication, negotiation and life skill development, *Qualitative Research in Sport & Exercise Psychology, 1*(1), 72-88.

Camire, M., Trudel, P., & Forneris, T. (2012). Coaching and transferring life skills: Philosophies and strategies used by model high school coaches. *The Sport Psychologist, 26*(2), 243-260.

Carreres-Ponsoda, F., Carbonell, A. E., Cortell-Tormo, J., Fuster-Lloret, V., & Andreu-Cabrera, E. (2012). The relationship between out-of-school sport participation and positive you development. *Journal of Human Sport & Exercise*, *7*(3), 671-683.

Coakley, J. (2011). Youth sports: What counts as "positive development?" *Journal of Sport & Social Issues*, *35*, 306-324.

Collins, K., Gould, D., Lauer, L., & Chung, Y. (2009). Coaching life skills through football: Philosophical beliefs of outstanding high school football coaches. *International Journal of Coaching Science, 3*(1), 1-26.

Danish, S. J. (2002a). *Going for the goal: Leader manual* (4 ed.), Richmond, VA: Life Skills Associates.

Danish, S. J. (2002b). *SUPER (Sports United to Promote Education and Recreation) program: Leader manual* (3rd ed.), Richmond: Life Skills Center, Virginia Commonwealth University.

Danish, S. J., & D'Augelli, A. R. (1983). *Helping skills II: Life development intervention.* New York, NY: Human Sciences.

Danish, S., Petitpas, A., & Hale, B. (1993). Life development interventions with athletes: Life skills through sports. *The Counseling Psychologist*, *21*, 352–385.

Danish, S. J., Taylor, T. E., & Fazio, R. J. (2003). Enhancing adolescent development through sports and leisure. In G. R. Adams & M. D. Berznsley (Eds.), *Blackwell Handbook of Adolescence* (pp. 92-108). Malden, MA: Blackwell Publishing.

Deci, E. L., & Ryan, R. M. (Eds.) (2002). *Handbook of self-determination research.* Rochester, NY: University of Rochester Press.

Deci, E., & Ryan, R. (2008). Facilitating optimal motivation and psychological well-being across life's domains. *Canadian Psychology, 49*, 14–23.

Duda, J. L., & Balaguer, I. (2007). Coach-created motivational climate. In S. Jowett & D. Lavallee (Eds.), *Social psychology of sport* (pp. 117-130). Champaign, IL: Human Kinetics.

Durlak, J. A., Weissberg, R. P., & Pachan, M. (2010). A meta-analysis of after-school programs that seek to promote personal and social skills in children and adolescents. *American Journal of Community Psychology, 45*, 294-309.

Dworkin, J. B., Larson, R., & Hansen, D. (2003). Adolescents' accounts of growth experiences in youth activities. *Journal of Youth and Adolescents, 32*(1), 17-26.

Eccles, J. S., & Barber, B. L. (1999). Student council, volunteering, basketball, or marching band: What kind of extracurricular involvement matters? *Journal of Adolescent Research, 14,* 10-43.

Eccles, J. S., Barber, B. L., Stone, M., & Hunt, J. (2003). Extracurricular activities and adolescent development. *The Journal of Social Issues, 59*, 865-889.

Flett, M. R., Gould, D., Griffes, K. R., & Lauer, L. (2012). The views of more versus less experienced coaches in underserved communities. *International Journal of Coaching Science, 6*(1), 3-26.

Flett, M. R., Gould, D., Griffes, K. R., & Lauer, L. (in press). Tough love for underserved youth: A comparison of more and less effective coaching. *The Sport Psychologist.*

Flett, M. R., Gould, D., & Lauer, L. (2012). A study of underserved youth sports program using the Youth Program Quality Assessment. *Journal of Applied Sport Psychology, 24*(3), 1-15.

Forneris, T., Camire, M., & Trudel, P. (2012). The development of life skills and values in high school sport: Is there a gap between stakeholder's expectations and perceived experiences? *International Journal of Sport & Exercise Psychology, 10*(1), 9-23.

Forneris, T., Danish, S. J., & Scott, D. L. (2007). Setting goals, solving problems, and seeking social support: Developing adolescents' abilities through a life skills program. *Adolescence, 42,*103-114.

Fry, M. D. (2010). Creating a positive climate for young athletes. *Journal of Sport Psychology in Action, 1*(1), 33-41.

Fry, M. D., & Gano-Overway, L. A. (2010). Exploring the contribution of the caring climate to the youth sports experience. *Journal of Applied Sport Psychology, 22*, 294-304.

Fry, M. D., Guivernau, M., Kim, M., Newton, M., Gano-Overway, L. A., & Magyar, T. M. (2011). Youth perspectives of a caring climate, emotional regulation, and psychological well-being. *Sport, Exercise & Performance Psychology, 9*(1), 44-57.

Gass, M. (1985). Programming the transfer of learning in adventure education. *Journal of Experiential Education, 8*(3), 18-24.

Goudas, M., Dermitzaki, I., Leondari, A., & Danish, S. J. (2006). The effectiveness of teaching a life skills program in a physical education context. *European Journal of Psychology of Education, 21*, 429-438.

Goudas, M., & Giannoudis, G. (2008). A team-sports-based life-skills program in a physical education context. *Learning & Instruction, 18*, 528-536.

Gould, D., & Carson, S. (2008). Life skills development through sport: Current status and future directions. *Sport & Exercise Psychology Reviews, 1,* 58-78.

Gould, D., & Carson, S. (2010). The relationship between perceived coaching behavior and developmental benefits of high school sports participation. *The Hellenic Journal of Psychology, 7,* 298-314.

Gould, D., & Carson, S. (2011). Young athletes perceptions of the relationship between coaching behaviors and developmental experiences. *International Journal of Coaching Science, 5*(2), 3-29.

Gould, D., Collins, K., Lauer, L., & Chung, Y. (2006). Coaching life skills: A working model. *Sport and Exercise Psychology Review, 2*(1), 10-18.

Gould, D., Collins, K., Lauer, L., & Chung, Y. (2007). Coaching life skills through football: A study of award winning high school coaches. *Journal of Applied Sport Psychology, 19*(1), 16-37.

Gould, D., Flett, M. R., & Lauer, L. (2012). The relationship between psychosocial developmental and the sports climate experienced by underserved youth. *Psychology of Sport & Exercise, 13*(1), 80-87.

Gould, D., Voelker, D. K., & Griffes, K. (2013). Best coaching practices for developing team captains. *The Sport Psychologist*, 27, 13-26.

Hansen, D. M., & Larson, R. (2007). Amplifiers of developmental and negative experiences in organized activities: Dosage, motivation, lead roles, and adult-youth ratios. *Journal of Applied Developmental Psychology, 28*, 360-374.

Hansen, D. M., Larson, R. W., & Dworkin, J. B. (2003). What adolescents learn in organized youth activities: A survey of self-reported developmental experiences. *Journal of Research on Adolescence, 13*, 25-55.

Hartmann, D., & Kwauk, C. (2011). Sport and development: An overview, critique, and reconstruction. *Journal of Sport & Social Issues, 35*(3), 284-305.

Hellison, D. (2011). *Teaching responsibility through physical activity* (3rd ed.). Champaign, IL: Human Kinetics.

Hellison, D. R., & Cutforth, N. (1997). Extended day programs for urban children and youth: From theory to practice. In H. Walberg, O. Reyes, & R. Weissberg (Eds.) *Urhan children and youth: Interdisciplinary perspectives, policies and programs* (pp. 223 249). San Francisco, CA: Jossey Bass.

Hellison, D., & Walsh, D. (2002). Responsibility-based youth programs evaluation: Investigating the investigations. *Quest, 54*, 292-307.

Hodge, K., Danish, S., & Martin, J. (2012). Developing a conceptual framework for life skills interventions. *The Counseling Psychologist, 41(8),* 1125-1152.

Holt, N., Tamminen, K. A., Tink, L., & Black, D. (2009). An interpretative analysis of life skills associated with sport participation. *Qualitative Research in Sport & Exercise, 1*(2), 160-175.

Holt, N., Tink, L., Mandigo, J. L., & Fox, K. R. (2008). Do youth learn life skills through their involvement in high school sport: A case study. *Canadian Journal of Education, 31*(2), 281-304.

Jones, M., & Lavallee, D. (2009). Exploring perceived like skills development and participation in sport. *Qualitative Research in Sport & Exercise, 1*(1), 36-50.

Kronspan, A. S. (2007). The early years of sport psychology: The work and influence of Pierre de Couberin. *Journal of Sport Behavior, 30*(1), 77-93.

Larson, R. (2000). Toward psychology of positive youth development, *American Psychologist, 55*(1), 170-183.

Larson, R. W. (2011). Positive development in a disorderly world. *Journal of Research on Adolescence, 21*(2), 317-334.

Larson, R. W., & Brown, J. R. (2007). Emotional development in adolescence: What can be learned from a high school theater program? *Child Development, 78*(4), 1083-1099.

Larson, R. W., Hansen, D. M., & Moneta, G. (2006). Differing profiles of developmental experiences across types of organized youth activities. *Developmental Psychology, 42*(5), 849-863.

Larson, R. W., & Walker, K. (2006). Learning about the "real world" in an urban arts program. *Journal of Adolescent Research, 21*, 244-268.

Li, W., Wright, P. M., Rukavina, P. B., & Pickering, M. (2008). Measuring students' perceptions of personal and social responsibility and the relationship to intrinsic motivation in urban physical education. *Journal of Teaching Physical Education, 27*, 167-178.

MacDonald, D. J., Côté, J., & Deakin, J. (2010). The impact of informal coach training on the personal development of youth sport athletes. *International Journal of Sports Science & Coaching, 5*(3), 363-372.

Mahoney, J. L., Vandell, D. L., Simpkins, S., & Zarrett, N. (2009). Adolescent out-of-school activities. In R. M. Lerner & L. Sternberg (Eds.), *Handbook of adolescent psychology* (Vol. 2, 3rd ed., pp. 228-267). Hoboken, NJ: Wiley.

Martinek, T., Schilling, T., & Johnson, D. (2001). Transferring personal and social responsibility of underserved youth to the classroom. *Urban Review, 33*(1), 29-45.

McCallister, S. G., Blinde, E. M., & Weiss, W. M. (2000). Teaching values and implementing philosophies: Dilemmas of the youth sport coach. *The Physical Educator, 57*, 34-45.

National Research Council and Institute of Medicine (2002). Community programs to promote youth development. In J. Eccles & J. A. Gootman (Eds.), *Board on children, youth and families, division of behavioral and social sciences and education.* Washington, DC: The National Academy Press.

O'Hearn, T., & Gatz, M. (1999). Evaluating a psychosocial competence program for urban adolescents. *Journal of Primary Prevention, 20*, 119–124.

O'Hearn, T., & Gatz, M. (2002). Going for the Goal: Improving youth's problem-solving skills through a school-based intervention. *Journal of Community Psychology, 30*, 281-303.

Papacharisis, V. P., Goudas, M., Danish, S. J., & Theodorakis, Y. (2005). The effectiveness of teaching a life skills program in a sport context. *Journal of Applied Sport Psychology, 17*(3), 247-254.

Petitpas, A. J., Cornelius, A. E., Van Raalte, J. L., & Jones, T. (2005). A framework for planning youth sport programs that foster psychosocial development. *The Sport Psychologist, 19*, 63-80.

Petitpas, A. J., Van Raalte. J. L., Cornelius. A. E., & Presbrey, J. (2004). A life skills development program for high school student athletes. *The Journal of Primary Care, 24*(3), 325-334.

Shields, D. L. L., & Bredemeier, B. L. (2007). Advances in sport morality research. In G. Tenenbaum & R. C. Eklund (Eds.), *Handbook of sport psychology* (3rd ed., pp. 662–684). Hoboken, NJ: Wiley & Sons.

Smith, R. E., Smoll, F. L., & Cummings, F. L. (2007). Effects of a motivational climate on intervention for coaches on youth athletes' sport performance anxiety. *Journal of Sport & Exercise Psychology, 29*(1), 39-59.

Strachan, L., Côté, J., & Deakin, J. (2009). "Specializers" versu*s "samplers" in youth sport: Comparing experiences and outcomes. The Sport Psychologist, 23*(1), 77-92.

Waldron, J. J. (2012). A social norms approach to hazing prevention workshops. *Journal of Sport Psychology in Action, 3*(1), 12-20.

Watson, D. L., Newton, M., & Kim, M. (2003). Recognition of values based constructs in a summer physical activity program. *Urban Review, 35*, 217-232.

Weiss, M. R. (Ed.) (2004). *Developmental sport and exercise psychology: A lifespan perspective*. Morgantown, WV: Fitness Information Technology.

Weiss, M. R. (2006). *The First Tee 2005 research summary: Longitudinal effects of the First Tee Life Skills Educational Program on positive youth development.* St. Augustine, FL: The First Tee.

Weiss, M. R. (2011). Teach the children well: A holistic approach to developing psychosocial and behavioral competencies through pe. *Quest, 63*(1), 55-65

Weiss, M. R., Smith, A. L., & Stuntz, C. P. (2008). Moral development in sport and physical activity: Theory, research, and intervention. In T. S. Horn (Ed.), *Advances in sport psychology* (3rd ed., pp. 187-210). Champaign, IL: Human Kinetics.

Weiss, M. R., Stuntz, C. P., Bhalla, J., Bolter, N. D., & Price, M. S. (2013). 'More than a game': Impact of the First Tee life skills development program on positive youth development: Project introduction and first year findings. *Qualitative Research in Sport, Exercise and Health*, *5*(2), 214-244.

Wells, M. S., & Arthur-Banning, S. G. (2008). The logic of youth development: Constructing a logic model of youth development through sport. *Journal of Parks and Recreation Administration*, *26*(2), 189-202.

Whitley, M. A., Bean, E. A., & Gould, D. R. (2011). On the fields of the Motor City: Underserved athletes' perceptions of their coaches. *Journal of Coaching Education, 4*(3), 97-125.

Wood, D., Larson, R. W., & Brown, J. R. (2009). How adolescents come to see themselves as more responsible through participation in youth. *Child Development*, *80*(1), 259-309.

Wright, P. M., & Burton, S. (2008). Promoting life skills through physical activity: A qualitative program evaluation. *Journal of Teaching Physical Education, 27*, 138-154.

W. K. Kellogg Foundation (2004). *Logic model development guide: using logic models to bring together planning, evaluation, and action*. Battle Creek, MI: Author.

In: Positive Human Functioning ... Volume 2 ISBN: 978-1-62948-973-5
Editors: A. R. Gomes, R. Resende and A. Albuquerque © 2014 Nova Science Publishers, Inc.

Chapter 5

HUMAN DEVELOPMENT PROGRAMMING: FOSTERING WELL-BEING THROUGHOUT ADULTHOOD

***Tanya Forneris*[1], *Tanya Halsall*[1], *Corliss Bean*[1] *and Steven J. Danish*[2]**
[1]School of Human Kinetics, University of Ottawa, Ottawa, Canada
[2]Department of Psychology, Virgnia Commonwealth University, Virginia, US

ABSTRACT

In the past few decades there has been an increased focus on positive human functioning. More specifically, in 2000 Seligman and Csikszentmihalyi outlined the importance of creating a shift in the field of psychology to focus on human strengths. They argued that the traditional focus of working to repair weaknesses is not an effective mechanism for helping individuals thrive or even prevent illness. This goal of this chapter is to provide an overview of how researchers and practitioners have come to understand and enhance positive human functioning throughout adulthood. Although the focus of this chapter is adulthood we begin with a brief overview of the transition period from youth to adulthood and briefly discuss whether positive outcomes typically associated with strength-based interventions, such as life skills programs, are maintained throughout adulthood. The second section discusses the young adulthood and the evidence indicating the need for continued opportunities to develop life skills as youth transition into this life stage. The third and fourth sections of the chapter focus on positive human functioning in middle adulthood and late adulthood, respectively. Overall, there are various ways in which researchers and practitioners have defined and work to enhance positive human functioning throughout the lifespan. From the research it is evident that interventions to foster such positive human functioning need to begin early in life and that these opportunities should be continually available throughout the lifespan as each stage of life presents new challenges. We hope that this chapter will help both researchers and practitioners to advance knowledge related to positive human functioning and develop increased opportunities to help individuals to live successful and fulfilling lives.

INTRODUCTION

In recent decades there has been an increased focus on positive human functioning. In 2000, the *American Psychologist* devoted a complete issue to the topic of positive psychology. The leading article introducing this issue was written by Seligman and Csikszentmihalyi (2000) who outlined the importance of creating a shift in the field of psychology to focus on human strengths. They argued that the traditional focus of reactive forms of interventions that worked to repair weaknesses is not an effective mechanism for helping individuals thrive or even prevent illness. Seligman and Csikszentmihalyi stated that the aim of positive psychology is "to begin to catalyze a change in the focus of psychology from preoccupation only with repairing the worst things in life to also building positive qualities" (2000, p. 5).

This chapter will provide an overview of how researchers and practitioners have worked to understand and enhance positive human functioning throughout adulthood. Although we have seen a shift within the larger psychology field towards a holistic development since the turn of the century, many researchers and practitioners have been using such an approach for many years. One such example is the Life Development Intervention (LDI) orientation proposed by Danish and colleagues in 1980 (Danish, Smyer, & Nowak, 1980). This orientation focuses on helping individuals develop capacity and competence in life planning so as to enable them to encounter and successfully manage both routine and unexpected life events. Although life events are often considered as discrete, the LDI orientation recognizes such events as processes that commence prior to the event and continue well after the event. Although the focus of this chapter is adulthood, we begin with a brief overview of the transition period from youth to adulthood. The remainder of the chapter will focus on three different stages of adulthood: young adulthood, middle adulthood and late adulthood. In each section we review the literature related to positive human functioning and the mechanisms by which researchers and practitioners can enhance positive functioning and well-being throughout these different stages of adulthood.

Within the field of developmental psychology, a number of prevention approaches emerged in the 70's and 80's that targeted youth (Catalano, Berglund, Ryan, Lonczak, & Hawkins, 2002). According to Catalano and colleagues (2002) these prevention approaches placed an emphasis on providing resources to support youth prior to the development of problem behavior (e.g., drug and alcohol use). However, starting in the late 80's a number of researchers began to criticize this approach as it was recognized by both researchers and practitioners that the typical prevention approach was not showing great levels of effectiveness (Catalano et al., 2002; Ennett, Tobler, Ringwalt, & Flewelling, 1994; Mitchell et al., 1997). In the 1990's there was a call from researchers to recognize that helping youth develop into successful adults requires more than avoiding problem behaviors (Danish & Nellen, 1997). As a result, a consensus began to develop that a successful transition to adulthood requires more than avoiding drugs, violence, or precocious sexual activity. The promotion of children's social, emotional, behavioral, and cognitive development began to be seen as key to enhancing development and preventing problem behaviors (W.T. Grant Consortium on the School-Based Promotion of Social Competence, 1992). These researchers advocated that an emphasis should be placed on the development of strengths (e.g., life skills) in key domains of functioning such as social, emotional, cognitive, and behavioral. For the purposes of this chapter we use the definition of life skills developed by Danish, Petitpas, and Hale (1993) which states that life skills are those skills that enables individuals to succeed in the different environments in which they live such as work, home and community. Life skills can be behavioural (e.g., communicating effectively), cognitive (e.g., effective decision making), interpersonal (e.g., being assertive) or intrapersonal (e.g., setting goals). It was believed that enhancing development in these areas would be the key in preventing problem behaviors and it was recognized that the idea of being "problem free is not fully prepared" (Pittman & Irby, 1996, p. 2) was critical in moving forward what is now known as the field of positive youth development (PYD).

In support of this growing consensus were the findings from the extensive review of 77 PYD programs by Catalano and colleagues (2002) that found that effective programs were those which focused on strengthening social, emotional, cognitive and/or behavioral competencies, self-efficacy, and family and community standards for healthy social and personal behaviors. It was also noted that 75% of the programs focused on enhancing relationships between youth and adults as well as increasing opportunities for participation in positive social activities. These programs showed a number of positive outcomes including, but not limited to better school attendance, increased academic achievement, enhanced decision making and interpersonal skills, self-efficacy, healthy peer and adult relationships, and decreased problem behaviors such as substance use, violence and risky sexual behavior. Two additional components that were present in the majority of programs was the use of a curriculum (96% of programs) and programs that were implemented for at least nine months (80% of programs).

As mentioned above, the overall goal of PYD programming is to enable youth to become successful and contributing adults (Danish, Forneris, Hodge, & Heke, 2004; Lerner, Almerigi, Theokas, & Lerner, 2005). However, adulthood still involves a number of transitions and as a result adults still face numerous challenges. Although we know that PYD programs can enhance various youth outcomes it is important to understand whether these outcomes will last over the course of adulthood and whether there is a need for ongoing interventions in adulthood to maintain and build upon these strengths and positive outcomes.

Are Positive Youth Outcomes Maintained in Adulthood?

There is some evidence that positive outcomes resulting from youth engagement in extracurricular and PYD programs are maintained in young adulthood. Roth and colleagues examined 15 different programs designed to help youth gain the competencies and knowledge they would need to meet the potential challenges they would face as they matured (Roth, Brooks-Gunn, Murray & Foster, 1998). The results of the study showed that programs of longer duration seemed to lead to cumulative positive outcomes with prolonged participation. In a more recent research, Mahoney, Cairns, and Farmer (2003) found a positive relationship between participation in school-based extracurricular activities and college attendance, particularly for youth with low interpersonal competence. Furthermore, researchers using data from the National Education Longitudinal Study in the United States found that consistent participation in organized programming throughout adolescence was associated with civic engagement and attending college (Zaff, Moore, Papillo, & Williams, 2003). Similarly, using data from the National Education Longitudinal Study, it was discovered that youth who participated in more organized activities for a longer duration (2 years or more) were more likely to exhibit higher educational achievement, civic engagement, and occupational success as young adults. These positive outcomes were maintained for as many as eight years after the completion of high school compared to those youth who were not involved at all or for as long (Gardner, Roth & Brooks-Gunn, 2008).

Unfortunately, there is a lack of longitudinal research to understand the lasting impact of youth engagement and PYD programs in adulthood. After high school many youth face the transition into post-secondary education. The next section of this chapter will examine the current research on the psychological well-being of university students and the need for life skills or strength-based programs to enhance the development of young adults.

POSITIVE HUMAN FUNCTIONING IN YOUNG ADULTHOOD

Entering into college or university is often seen as the time when adolescents transition into adulthood. However, this time can constitute a stressful transition for many students. To graduate from college or university students often have to persevere through a number of psychosocial stressors such as moving away from home, increased workload, decreased financial resources, increased academic responsibilities and pressure to perform, establishing new social networks, and adapting to increased independence. In recent years, particularly in North America, research has indicated that university students report higher levels of psychological distress and seek mental health services in greater numbers than in years previous. Watkins, Hunt, and Eisenberg (2012) found that mental health concerns for which students present to counselling centers vary greatly. These concerns include typical challenges experienced during this life transition such as stress and anxiety to severe mental disorders such as major depression and schizophrenia. In the United States, an assessment of college health was conducted in 2008 and the results indicated that more than 30% of undergraduate students reported feeling depressed to the point of impacting their daily functioning at some point during the academic year (American College Health Association, 2009; Watkins et al., 2012). In other research it was found that the number of undergraduate students who have been diagnosed with depression has increased between 10-15% since the early 2000's (Gallagher, 2008) and that 10% reported at least one episode of suicidal ideation (Drum, Brownson, Burton Denmark, & Smith, 2009). Similar findings are also true for campuses across Canada. In 2011, the Centre for Student Development at Ryerson University experienced a 200% increase in the demand for students presenting in crisis (Lunau, 2012). Similarly, at the University of Alberta over 50% of students reported feeling hopeless and/or overwhelming anxiety in the past year and 7% reported seriously considering suicide (Lunau, 2012).

This increase in mental health difficulties has naturally led to an increased demand for mental health services on campus which has placed a strain on the existing resources in counselling centers. According to a National Survey of Counseling Center Directors (2009) there is typically only one counselor for every 1,527 students (Gallagher, 2010). In Canada, the ratio of students to counselors is similar. For example, Lunau (2012) reported that Ryerson only has 19 full time staff (family physicians, psychologists and counselors) and one part time staff (psychiatrist) for 28,300 students. Furthermore, Watkins et al. (2012) and Gallagher (2008) found that counseling center administrators are experiencing increased concerns related to meeting the mental health demands of students such as staff burnout, staff shortages during peak times (e.g., exams, end of semester), a decrease in the ability to provide adequate focus on students presenting with severe difficulties, and the need to end treatment for students prematurely to be able to keep up with demand.

As a result, numerous students have not been able to access the resources they need to cope effectively and counseling centers are experiencing high levels of workload and burnout. Therefore, researchers (Watkins et al., 2012; Wood, 2012) have advocated for increased avenues and/or resources to help students develop the skills needed to effectively manage this life transition. We argue that a focus on developing life skills is warranted given that research has shown that individual factors are stronger predictors compared to institutional factors for experiencing mental health difficulties (Byrd & McKinney, 2012). Moreover, research has found that coping abilities is the individual factor that had the strongest influence on mental health, while perceptions of the campus climate and overall satisfaction with the college/university significantly predicts positive mental health. As a result, it is important to ensure students have the opportunity to develop life skills and that campuses work to increase the levels of social support students experience during this life transition.

One possible mechanism for increasing students' life skills would be the addition of courses or initiatives designed to develop such skills. Some universities and colleges have begun to integrate courses of this nature. For example, in Canada a large college located in Southern Ontario offers two courses in life skills development while a university located in Eastern Ontario has incorporated a course on enhancing quality living skills. In addition, in Hong Kong, Dr. Daniel Shek has developed a course that focuses on holistic development of students which will be discussed in greater detail below. Although examples of such life skill courses have begun to appear across college and university campuses there is controversy over whether such courses are "academic enough" for the typical curriculum. The ongoing debate seems to be whether such programming should be integrated into the actual curriculum or offered as a non-academic service or program. The greatest benefit of integrating such programs into actual curriculum would be that all students would have the opportunity to develop the life skills that could enable them to cope more effectively with the increased demands experienced during this life transition. The strongest argument against embedding such programming is that it takes time away from learning content-specific knowledge. However, in debating this issue it may be important to return to arguments put forth by Harward (2007).

Harward argued that original purposes of liberal education, on which post-secondary education was built, are often ignored by our present day institutions. Harward described three overarching purposes of liberal education which include the *epistemic* which involves the coming to know, discovery, and the advancing of knowledge and understanding, the *eudemonic* which involves the fuller realization of the learner meaning the actualizing of the person's potential to achieve individual well-being and happiness, and the *civic* which focuses on helping an individual understand the 'other' and the responsibility that comes from community and civic engagement. Such engagement allows for both open inquiry and self-realization. It is argued that our current institutions place a strong focus on the epistemic purpose at the expense of the others. As a result, research has shown that between 40-60% of students are disengaged from their academic experiences and this disengagement is often expressed through alcohol and drug abuse, depressive symptoms and suicide (Blum & Libby, 2004).

Unfortunately, most post-secondary institutions have often dealt with issues related to student disengagement by providing treatment (such as counseling services) using a medical model. Moreover, institutions often ask the student to leave the institution due to concerns of liability. Little effort has been put forth to integrate strength-based programs into the curriculum which, as mentioned above, would provide learning opportunities to help students develop a variety of life skills. These life skills could help fulfill the eudemonic and civic purposes of education which in turn could foster well-being of students. In response to this current climate, Harward created the Bringing Theory to Practice project. The overall objective of this project is to assist institutions to provide all three purposes of education. Harward identified service learning and community-based research as ideal initiatives as they actively engage students and therefore have the potential to change the attitudes, behaviors, and dispositions of students. Both service learning and community-based research also necessitate an academic focus which results in students taking a more active role in their learning process, taking on greater responsibility, and understanding that not all learning takes place in the classroom.

In 2012, the Bringing Theory to Practice program provided funding to 61 institutions to assist them in integrating initiatives to enhance the relationship between civic engagement, psychosocial well-being, and engaged learning. Although evaluation of these initiatives have yet to be published, past research has shown that service learning leads to increased academic motivation, attitudes towards education, grade point average, motivation to volunteer, and enhanced moral development (Conway, Amel, & Gerwein, 2009). Moreover, research has shown that service learning helped students recognize that people, such as themselves, can make a difference, that leadership and volunteering experiences are important activities, the need for equal opportunities for everyone, increased positive perceptions toward co-workers, recognition of multiple viewpoints or perspectives, increased civic awareness, greater resolve or sense of persistence even when the ability to succeed was unknown, increased pro-social decision making, increased pro-social reasoning and identity exploration (Batchelder & Root, 1994; Conway et al., 2009; Giles & Eyler, 1994).

As mentioned above, another initiative created to help enhance human functioning of university students has been the development of a positive youth development course by Dr. Daniel Shek for university students at the Hong Kong Polytechnic University entitled "Tomorrow's Leaders" (Shek & Sun, 2012). Similar to Harward's (2007) Bringing to Theory to Practice program, this course was developed in response to the lack of programs aimed at the holistic development of university students. Shek and Sun discussed how there is a plethora of such programs targeting high school students, but a lack of such resources for young adults. Research evaluating the "Tomorrow's Leaders" course have examined the impact of the course and found that students showed a number of positive outcomes including increases in resilience, social competence, emotional competence, cognitive competence, behavioral competence, moral competence, self-determination, self-efficacy, prosocial norms, and belief in the future. Furthermore, over 90% of the students provided a positive evaluation of the course and 94% believed that the course had a positive impact on their lives (Shek & Sun, 2012).

Overall, the research indicates that the transition into young adulthood can lead to increased distress and there appears to be a lack of opportunities available for students to develop life skills needed to effectively meet the various demands of this transitional phase. Given the promising outcomes related to the integration of service learning as well as courses focused on helping students develop life skills it is recommended that individuals involved in working with young adults, particularly those in post-secondary institutions where the majority of young adults spend their time, return to a focus on the original purpose of liberal education which involves a balanced focus on gaining knowledge, enhancing well-being, and civic engagement. Such a balanced focus will lead to increased positive functioning and also help individuals be able to successfully negotiate the challenges they will face in middle adulthood.

Positive Human Functioning in Middle Adulthood

Research concerning middle adulthood has not focused on life skills programs per se, however, there has been a substantial amount of research on well-being. Interventions designed to enhance well-being during this stage of life are often termed strength-based interventions. Sin and Lyubomirsky (2009) defined strength-based or positive psychology interventions as "treatment methods or intentional activities aimed at cultivating positive feelings, positive behaviors, or positive cognitions" (p. 467).

Systematic research reviews of strength-based interventions have shown positive effects on well-being. Sin and Lyubomirsky conducted a meta-analysis of 51 such interventions and found that these interventions significantly enhanced well-being and decreased depressive symptoms. In another study, Mitchell and colleagues found that strength-based interventions showed increases in subjective well-being (Mitchell, Stanimirovic, Klein, & Vella-Brodrick, 2009). Moreover, Gander and colleagues examined the impact of several strength-based interventions and found that eight out of nine demonstrated an increase on participant happiness and that all of the interventions led to decreased depression (Gander, Proyer, Ruch, & Wyss, 2012).

In adulthood, strength-based interventions vary in how they are implemented. Two common forms of implementing such programs are in the workplace and more recently via the internet. The rationale for such forms of implementation is that the workplace and internet can reach large numbers of adults in ways that make it convenient as they provide easy accessibility. Below is an overview of some examples of both workplace and internet strength-based interventions.

The first example is a resilience building program called 'Promoting Adult Resilience' (PAR; Millear, Liossis, Shochet, Biggs, & Donald, 2008). This program is a strength-based resilience program that integrates interpersonal and cognitive-behavioral therapy perspectives from psychology. The program is implemented in the workplace and is designed to draw on everyday examples of workplace situations and work-life balance issues. PAR was based on the Resourceful Adolescent Program (RAP; Shochet et al., 2001) which is a school-based program that has shown to be effective in reducing depression, increasing regulation of affect, improving cognitive and attribution styles, and improving interpersonal relationships (Shochet et al., 2001; Shochet & Ham, 2004). The PAR program is typically implemented by a psychologist to small groups of individuals ($N = 8$ to 14 people) and uses program manuals and workbooks to present the program material. The sessions of the program cover a number of areas of positive functioning including understanding personal strengths and resilience, managing stress, challenging and changing self-talk, problem solving work-life problems, preventing and managing conflict. The last session of the program provides an overall summary of the program and skills taught throughout the program.

An evaluation of an 11-week implementation of the PAR program that involved 150 participants showed that the PAR group compared to a non-intervention matched group improved significantly in coping self-efficacy and stress, reported decreased depressive symptoms, and greater work-life balance. Moreover, these effects were maintained at a six month follow-up (Millear et al., 2008). In another evaluation of PAR, Liossis, Shochet, Millear, and Biggs (2009) found similar results even though the program took place over the course of only seven weeks. The intervention group showed significant improvements in coping self-efficacy, work satisfaction, and work-life balance. In addition, the program participants reported an increased positive outlook in their work and personal lives, as well as improved relationships with their colleagues in the program.

As mentioned above, the internet is a growing medium for the implementation of strength-based programs for adults. As a result, the number of internet interventions available for adults to help enhance positive functioning has been growing rapidly. One example of the use of the internet for enhancing well-being in adulthood is the intervention conducted by Seligman, Steen, Park, and Peterson (2005). More specifically, Seligman and colleagues used the internet for participant recruitment, data collection, and intervention delivery. In this one-week intervention, participants were randomly assigned to one of five happiness intervention exercises or a placebo control group. The five intervention exercises were labelled: (1) *a gratitude visit* which involved participants writing a letter of gratitude to someone in their life; (2) *identifying three good things in life* which involved the participants writing down three things that went well each day and a causal explanation for each good thing; (3) *identifying a time when the participant is at his/her best* which involved the participants writing about a time they were at their best and were asked to identify personal strengths during this time; (4) *identifying signature strengths* which involved the participants completing an inventory of character strengths and receiving feedback about their top five strengths; and (5) *identifying and using signature strengths* which involved identifying signature strengths as outlined above and then being asked to use their top five strengths in a new and different way every day for a week. The placebo control group participants were simply asked to write about their earliest memories for a period of one week. The participants received instructions for their assigned activity via email and were encouraged to contact the researchers with any questions they had about their activity.

Results of the intervention evaluation indicated that two groups (identifying three good things in life and identifying and using signature strengths in a new way) showed significant increases in overall happiness and decreases in depressive symptoms. These changes also persisted over a period of six months. In addition, individuals in the gratitude visit group showed improvements in happiness and decreases in depression, but these results were only maintained for a period of one month.

Although this intervention was internet-based, the intervention itself only took place over a one week period and there were no interactive web-based activities as everything was emailed to participants. As a result, Mitchell et al. (2009) built upon Seligman and colleagues (2005) intervention to examine the efficacy of a positive psychology internet-based intervention. Mitchell compared three groups (N = 160). One group received a strengths intervention, one group received a problem-solving intervention and the third group represented a placebo condition. A randomized controlled trial design was used to compare these three groups. The two intervention programs were delivered over three sessions, with a recommended 1-week break between sessions, and automated weekly email reminders to complete the next session. The strengths intervention was based on the identifying and using your strengths intervention developed by Seligman and colleagues. In the first session of this intervention, participants identified and prioritized their perceived strengths from a list of 24 signature strengths developed by Peterson and Park (2004). At the end of the session the participants were asked to share with a friend what they had learned about identifying their personal strengths. In the second session, participants provided feedback regarding their experience sharing with a friend what they had learned and then selected three of their top 10 strengths to further develop in their daily life. Participants were asked to practice their identified strengths and were provided an online journal diary to help them record their progress. The final session of the intervention focused on reviewing the progress the participant had made and summarized the information provided in the previous two sessions.

The problem solving intervention was based on a cognitive-behavioral approach and introduced participants to a six-step approach. The six steps include: (1) identify the problem; (2) generate possible solutions; (3) evaluate the alternatives; (4) decide on a solution; (5) implement the solution; and (6) evaluate and review progress. In the first session, participants were introduced to the first three steps to problem solving and at the end of the session participants were asked to share what they had learned about problem solving with a friend. At the beginning of the second session the participants were asked to provide feedback on the sharing activity they had completed and the rest of the session focused on the fourth and fifth steps which the participants were asked to apply to a real life problem. The participants were also provided an online the sixth step of the model and were given a summary of the complete six-step process.

The placebo control group was an abbreviated version of the problem solving intervention, but without utilizing any of the interactive web features. Unlike the problem solving group, participants were not asked to apply the problem solving information to a real life problem, nor were they asked to complete any offline tasks such as sharing what they learned with a friend. Results of an evaluation of this internet-based program showed that those in the strengths group reported increases in well-being, engagement and pleasure, while the problem solving group showed no significant changes and the placebo group actually showed decreases from pre to post program.

According to Mitchell et al. (2009):

Internet delivery of well-being interventions addresses many of the limitations of traditional approaches, in particular the internet provides a more accessible, sustainable, and personalised approach to health promotion than has previously been possible. Combining what is known from positive psychology and well-being research with internet intervention research offers an immense opportunity to develop the field of health promotion worldwide (p. 758).

In addition, a number of researchers have argued that programs designed to foster positive human functioning, such as the examples provided above, need to occur over the lifespan as programs with longer duration have been found to have better outcomes related to well-being (Roth et al., 1998; Seligman et al., 2005; Sin & Lyubomirsky, 2009). Therefore, although the transition into middle adulthood may not be as stressful as the transition into young adulthood there is a great need for strength-based programs. These programs would provide adults the opportunity to learn new or enhance existing life skills to help manage the multiple roles and demands individuals in this phase of life often face such as work, family, community involvement, and leisure time activities. It can also be argued that learning or strengthening such life skills will not only help enhance functioning during this life stage, but will also help in the transition into late adulthood.

POSITIVE HUMAN FUNCTIONING IN LATE ADULTHOOD

This section of the chapter discusses another common life transition often experienced in later adulthood: retirement. Retirement historically has signified the transition from an active work career to a life of leisure. This transition involves changes in perceptions, expectations, and priorities for the use of one's time and energies. Life events or transitions such as retirement can be viewed in two ways: as markers and as processes. When events are viewed as markers, they become milestones or transition points, giving shape and direction to the various aspects of a person's life (Neugarten & Hagestad, 1976). Some researchers assert that it is inappropriate, however, to consider events as solely markers that occur at single points in time (Danish et al., 1980). Events are also processes. They have histories of their own from the time they are anticipated, through their occurrences, until their aftermaths have been determined and assessed (Danish et al., 1980). It is this process that the marker signifies, but does not help describe. Viewing events only as markers underestimates the importance of the *context* of events. Events such as retirement do not occur in a vacuum; they occur in a rich life space of the individual, including competing demands from a variety of areas (e.g., work, family life, physical development) and people significant to the individual (Danish et al., 1980). There are also other factors that affect the retirement process as well. The timing of the event is critical. Retiring in one's 30's, 40's or early 50's like athletes and military members do is much different than retiring at 65. The more "on time" retirement is, the greater the likelihood that both informal and formal support networks will exist to ease or assist the change (Danish et al., 1980). Furthermore, when events are viewed as processes, rather than discrete occurrences, "event duration" includes the anticipation of the event, the event itself, and the post-event influences (Nowak, 1979). Many life events are anticipated before their actual occurrence and retirement is one such event and it offers sufficient opportunity for a "preoccurrence priming" that can serve to ease the transition into postoccurrence life. Finally, the probability of an event occurring impacts how it is perceived. High probability events such as retirement at 65 may receive much more support than low probability events such as retirement at 35 (Danish et al., 1980).

Research on retirement has primarily focused on understanding this transition as well as examining how well individuals adjust to this transition (Wang & Shultz, 2010). Wang, Henkens, and van Solinge (2011) argued that retirement represents a longitudinal process and throughout this process an individual's level of adjustment may fluctuate based on the resources available to that individual. They proposed a resource-based dynamic perspective to understand how individuals adjust to retirement. Wang et al. argued that the resource-based dynamic perspective is consistent with the balance of resources to deficits approach often used by researchers to understand how individuals adapt to a variety of life transitions.

Therefore, the adaption to a life transition, such as a retirement, depends on the ratio of resources to deficits, the individual's sense of competency, well-being, and health (Schlossberg, 1981). Wang et al. explain that if throughout retirement retirees total resources do not change significantly, meaning that individuals are able to maintain their lifestyle and activities, they may not experience significant changes in adjustment whereas if an individual's resources decrease such as a loss in income or a decreased ability to engage in the activities they enjoy there may be a negative impact on adjustment. In addition, Wang et al., also discussed how if retirement allows an individual to experience a gain in resources (e.g., gaining cognitive resources that were occupied by a stressful job or increasing amount of time spend in enjoyable activities), he or she may experience a positive change in adjustment level.

The resource-based dynamic perspective also presents a variety of antecedents that can influence the level of resources in the adjustment process, including variables from the macro level (e.g., social norms and government programs) the organizational level (human resources programs, climate of workplace), the job level (working conditions, attachment to the job), the household level (quality of relationships with significant others, caregiving demands), and the individual level (health behaviors, psychological well-being; Wang et al., 2011). Overall the literature is mixed with regards to how individuals typically cope during the transition into retirement. Some research has found individuals have a negative outlook regarding retirement and that such individuals can report greater depression and loneliness, lower life satisfaction and happiness, lower activity levels, increases in illness, difficulties with mobility, and decreases in mental health during retirement (Dave, Rashad, & Spasojevic, 2008; Kim & Moen, 2002; Richardson & Kilty, 1991). While other research has indicated that many people, particularly those looking forward to retirement, report enjoying this transition (Calasanti, 1996; Dorfman, 1992). As well, research has found that for some individuals retirement could be characterized as a benign event with neither a positive or negative impact on well-being (Gall, Evans, & Howard, 1997; Wu, Tang, & Yan, 2005). To help understand the differences, Wang and Bodner (2007) analyzed longitudinal data and found that over the course of eight years within the retirement process the majority of individuals (70%) do not experience any change to their well-being whereas a minority of individuals experience a negative impact on their well-being (approximately 25%) or a positive impact on their well-being (approximately 5%).

Wang and Shultz (2010) assert that these differences in experiences with retirement reflect the importance of recognizing the value of the dynamic nature of this transition and that researchers and practitioners need to work together to develop interventions to ensure that individuals positively adjust to the retirement. Unfortunately, very little research has led to development and/or evaluation of interventions designed to assist individuals during this transition. However, researchers have developed an understanding of the factors that can either positively or negatively impact the transition to retirement. We will provide of an overview of these factors and then discuss recommendations for the development of retirement interventions.

The factors that impact the transition to retirement are numerous but have been summarized in a number of categories such as individual attributes, preretirement job-related variables, family-related variables, retirement transition- related variables, and postretirement activities (Wang et al., 2011; Wang & Shultz, 2010). Individual attribute factors shown to be related to the retirement transition can include physical health, mental health, and financial status (Kim & Feldman, 2000; Pinquart & Schindler, 2007; van Solinge & Henkens, 2008; Wang, 2007). Pre-retirement job-related variables include work stress, job challenges, job dissatisfaction, unemployment before retirement, and work role identity (Pinquart & Schindler, 2007; Reitzas & Mutran, 2004; van Solinge & Henkens, 2008; Wang, 2007). Family-related variables include marital status and quality, number of dependent children, spouse working status, and losing a spouse during the transition (Kim & Feldman, 2000; Pinquart & Schindler, 2007; Szinovacz & Davey, 2004; van Solinge & Henkens, 2008; Wang, 2007). Retirement-transition variables include voluntariness of the retirement decision and retirement planning (Reitzas & Mutran, 2004; van Solinge & Henkens, 2008; Wang, 2007) and post-retirement activities include bridge employment, volunteer work and leisure activities (Dorfman & Douglas, 2006; Kim & Feldman, 2000; Wang, 2007; Zhan, Wang, Liu, & Schultz, 2009).

Researchers and practitioners involved in developing interventions to help individuals transition into retirement need to take these factors into consideration, but it is also recommended that retirement interventions adopt an enhancement, life-planning approach. Enhancement interventions are directed toward aiding individuals to embrace the future so that events provide opportunities for growth. In addition, in enhancement interventions the end state does not relate to a specific outcome, rather it focuses on the process which means that individuals develop the skills and abilities that enable them to plan for a variety of future life events (Danish & D'Augelli, 1980). An enhancement intervention has the following attributes: (a) a central focus on life events; (b) a developmental as opposed to a disease conception; and (c) a belief that experiencing past life events helps one prepare for future life events (Danish & D'Augelli, 1980).

It is recommended that those working with individuals to prepare for retirement use an enhancement approach for several reasons. First, proponents of enhancement interventions recognize that retirement must be considered as a process. Retirement is not simply the day at age 65 or 70 when one stops working; it is a process that can and should begin long before the transition out of the workforce. Second, enhancement interventions make specific assumptions regarding the competencies of individuals. Such interventions assume that individuals have both skills and deficits, and that they are to be active problem solvers and participants in the intervention (Kahn, 1975; Smyer & Gatz, 1979). Therefore, using an enhancement approach allows an individual to be involved in the process and encourages self-reliance and life planning so that they feel competent and empowered when making this transition. Third, the enhancement orientation decreases the need for professional personnel to have to intervene. In the late 1950's Albee (1959) pointed out the impossibility of training enough direct service personnel for the population in need of mental health services. A similar argument can be made for the personnel situation in the area of aging in general, and retirement in particular. Therefore, one strategy is to develop enhancement approaches that will reduce or minimize the reliance upon professional services. Fourth, as mentioned above, an enhancement orientation begins long before the active event of retirement and therefore involves much life-planning. In addition to making retirement a more positive experience, one's life satisfaction may improve across a number of life dimensions when individuals engage in life planning.

Conclusion

In sum, there are various ways in which researchers and practitioners have defined and work to enhance positive human functioning throughout the lifespan. The goal of this chapter was to provide an overview of the empirical evidence as well as provide examples of the types of programming that can be used to help individuals develop the necessary life skills that will enable them to live happy and successful lives. From the research it is evident that interventions to foster such positive human functioning need to begin early in life and that these opportunities need to be continually available throughout the lifespan as each stage of life presents new challenges. We hope that this chapter will help or inspire both researchers and practitioners to continue to advance knowledge to understand the factors that relate to positive human functioning. We also hope that such advances in knowledge lead to the development of more effective interventions designed to enhance functioning throughout the lifespan.

References

Albee, G. W. (1959). *Mental health manpower needs*. New York: Basic Books.

American College Health Association (2009). American College Health Association National College Health Assessment (ACHA–NCHA) spring 2008 reference group data report (abridged). *Journal of American College Health 54*, 201-211.

Batchelder, T. H., & Root, S. (1994). Effects of an undergraduate program to integrate academic learning and service: Cognitive, prosocial cognitive, and identity outcomes. *Journal of Adolescence, 17*, 341-355.

Blum, R. W., & H. Libby (2004). Executive summary. *Journal of School* Health *74*(7), 229-32.

Byrd, D. R., & McKinney, K. J. (2012). Individual, interpersonal and institutional level factors associated with the mental health of college students. *Journal of American College Health, 60*(3), 201-211.

Calasanti, T. M. (1996). Gender and life satisfaction in retirement: An assessment of the male model. *Journal of Gerontology: Social Sciences, 51B*, S18-S29.

Catalano, R. F., Berglund, M. L., Ryan, J. A. M., Lonczak, H. S., & Hawkins, J. D. (2002). Positive youth development in the United States: Research findings on evaluations of positive youth development programs. *The annals of the American academy of political and social science, 591*(1), 98-124.

Conway, J., Amel, E., & Gerwein, D. (2009). Teaching and learning in the social context: A meta-analysis of service learning's effects on academic, personal, social, and citizenship outcomes. *Teaching of Psychology, 36*, 233-245.

Danish, S. J., & D'Augelli, A. R. (1980). Promoting competence and enhancing development through life development intervention. In L. A. Bond & J. C. Rosen (Eds.), *Primary Prevention of Psychopathology* (Vol. 4, pp. 105-129). Hanover, N.H.: University Press of New England.

Danish, S. J., Forneris, T., Hodge, K., & Heke, I. (2004). Enhancing youth development through sport. *World Leisure Journal, 46*(3), 38-49.

Danish, S. J., & Nellen, V. C. (1997). New roles for sport psychologists: Teaching life skills through sport to at-risk youth. *Quest, 49*(1), 100-113.

Danish, S. J., Petitpas, A. J., & Hale, B. D. (1993). Life development intervention for athletes: Life skills through sports. *The Counseling Psychologist, 21*(3), 352-385.

Danish, S. J., Smyer, M. A., & Nowak, C. A. (1980). Developmental intervention: Enhancing life-event processes. *Life Span Development and Behavior, 3*, 339-366.

Dave, D., Rashad, I., & Spasojevic, J. (2008). The effects of retirement on physical and mental health outcomes. *Southern Economic Journal, 75*, 497-523.

Dorfman, L. T. (1992). Academics and the transition to retirement. *Educational Gerontology, 18*, 343–363.

Dorfman, L. T., & Douglas, K. (2005). Leisure and the retired professor: Occupational matters. *Educational Gerontology, 31*, 343-361.

Drum, D. J., Brownson, C., Burton, D. A., & Smith, S. E. (2009). New data on the nature of suicidal crises in college students: Shifting the paradigm. *Professional Psychology: Research and Practice 40*(3), 213-222.

Ennett, S. T., Tobler, N. S., Ringwalt, C. L., & Flewelling, R. L. (1994). How effective is drug abuse resistance education? A meta-analysis of Project DARE outcome evaluations. *American Journal of Public Health, 84*(9), 1394-1401.

Gall, T. L., Evans, D. R., & Howard, J. (1997). The retirement adjustment process: Changes in the well-being of male retirees across time. *Journal of Gerontology: Psychological Sciences, 52B*, P110-P117.

Gallagher, R. (2008). *National survey of counseling center directors 2008*. Retrieved February 16, 2013 from http://www.iacsinc.org/2008%20National%20Survey%20of%20Counseling%20Center%20Directors.pdf.

Gallagher, R. P. (2010). *National survey of counseling center directors: 2010*. International Association of Counseling Centers, Monograph 85. Retrieved February 16, 2013 from http://www.iacsinc.org/NSCCD%202010.pdf.

Gander, F., Proyer, R. T., Ruch, W., & Wyss, T. (2012). Strength-based positive interventions: Further evidence for their potential in enhancing well-being and alleviating depression. *Journal of Happiness Studies*, 1-19.

Gardner, M., Roth, J., & Brooks-Gunn, J. (2008). Adolescents' participation in organized activities and developmental success 2 and 8 years after high school: Do sponsorship, duration, and intensity matter? *Developmental Psychology, 44*(3), 814-830.

Giles, D. E., & Eyler, J. (1994). The impact of a college community service laboratory on students' personal, social, and cognitive outcomes. *Journal of Adolescence, 17*(4), 327-339.

Harward, D. (2007). Engaged learning and the core purposes of liberal education. *Liberal Education, 93*(1), 6-15.

Kahn, R. L. (1975). The mental health system and the future aged. *Gerontologist, 15*, 24-31.

Kim, J. E., & Moen, P. (2002). Retirement transitions, gender, and psychological well-being: A life-course, ecological model. *Journal of Gerontology: Psychological Sciences, 57B*, P212-P222.

Kim, S., & Feldman, D. C. (2000). Working in retirement: The antecedents of bridge employment and its consequences for quality of life in retirement. *Academy of Management Journal, 43*, 1195-1210.

Lerner, R. M., Almerigi, J. B., Theokas, C., & Lerner, J. V. (2005). Positive youth development. *Journal of Adolescence, 25*(1), 10-16.

Liossis, P. L., Shochet, I. M., Millear, P. M., & Biggs, H. (2009). The promoting adult resilience (PAR) program: The effectiveness of the second, shorter pilot of a workplace prevention program. *Behaviour Change, 26*(2), 97-112.

Lunau, K. (2012). The mental health on campus. *Macleans.* Retrieved from http://oncampus.macleans.ca/education/2012/09/05/the-mental-health-crisis-on-campus.

Mahoney, J. L., Cairns, B. D., & Farmer, T. W. (2003). Promoting interpersonal competence and educational success through extracurricular activity participation. *Journal of Educational Psychology, 95,* 409-418.

Millear, P. M., Liossis, P., Shochet, I. M. Biggs, H. C., & Donald, M. (2008). Being on PAR: outcomes of a pilot trial to improve mental health and wellbeing in the workplace with the Promoting Adult Resilience (PAR) Program. *Behaviour Change, 25*(4), 215-228.

Mitchell, D. A., Thomas, B. H., Devlin, M. C., Goldsmith, C. H., Willan, A., Singer, J., Marks, S., Watters, D., & Hewson, S. (1997). Evaluation of an educational program to prevent adolescent pregnancy. *Health Education and Behavior, 24*(3), 300-312.

Mitchell, J., Stanimirovic, R., Klein, B., & Vella-Brodrick, D. (2009). A randomized placebo controlled trial of a self-guided internet intervention promoting well-being. *Computers in Human Behavior, 25,* 749-760.

Neugarten, B., & Hagestad, G. (1976). Age and the life course. In R. H. Binstock & E. Shanas (Eds.), *Handbook of aging and the social sciences* (pp. 35-55). New York, NY: Van Nostrand Reinhold.

Nowak, C. (1979). *Life events research: Conceptual consideration.* Unpublished manuscript. Pennsylvania State University.

Peterson, C., & Park, N. (2004). Classification and measurement of character strengths: Implications for practice. In P. A. Linley & S. Joseph (eds.), *Positive psychology in practice* (pp.433-446). Hoboken, NJ: John Wiley & Sons.

Pinquart, M., & Schindler, I. (2007). Changes of life satisfaction in the transition to retirement: A latent-class approach. *Psychology and Aging, 22,* 442-455.

Pittman, K. J., & Irby, M. (1996). *Preventing problems or promoting development: Competing priorities or inseparable goals* [Online]. Available: http://www.iyf.org.

Reitzes, D. C., & Mutran, E. J. (2004). The transition into retirement: Stages and factors that influence retirement adjustment. *International Journal of Aging and Human Development, 59,* 63-84.

Richardson, V., & Kilty, K. M. (1991). Adjustment to retirement: Continuity vs. discontinuity. *International Journal of Aging and Human Development, 33,* 151-169.

Roth, J., Brooks-Gunn, J., Murray, L., & Foster, W. (1998). Promoting healthy adolescents: Synthesis of youth development program evaluations. *Journal of Research on Adolescence, 8*(4), 423-459.

Schlossberg, N. K. (1981). A model for analyzing human adaptation to transition. *The Counseling Psychologist, 9,* 2-18.

Seligman, M. E. P., & Csikszentmihalyi, M. (2000). Positive psychology: An introduction. *American Psychologist, 55,* 5-14.

Seligman, M. E. P., Steen, T., Park, N., & Peterson, C. (2005). Positive psychology progress: Empirical validation of interventions. *American Psychologist, 60*(5), 410-421.

Shek, D. T. L., & Sun, R. C. F. (2012). Promoting leadership and intrapersonal competence in university students: What can we learn from Hong Kong? *International Journal on Disability and Human Development, 11*(3), 221-228.

Shochet, I. M., Dadds, M. R., Holland, D., Whitefield, K., Harnett, P. H., & Osgarby, S. M. (2001). The efficacy of a universal school-based program to prevent adolescent depression. *Journal of Clinical Child Psychology, 30*(3), 303-315.

Shochet, I. M., & Ham, D. (2004). Universal school-based approaches to preventing adolescent depression: Past findings and future directions of the Resourceful Adolescent Program. *International Journal of Mental Health Promotion, 6*(3), 17-25.

Sin, N. L., & Lyubomirsky, S. (2009). Enhancing well-being and alleviating depressive symptoms with positive psychology interventions: A practice-friendly meta-analysis. Journal of Clinical *Psychology, 65*(5), 467-487.

Smyer, M. A., & Gatz, M. (1979). Aging and mental health: Business as usual? *American Psychologist, 34*, 240-246.

Szinovacz, M. E., & Davey, A. (2004). Honeymoons and joint lunches: Effects of retirement and spouse's employment on depressive symptoms. *Journal of Gerontology: Psychological Sciences, 59B*, P233-P245.

van Solinge, H., & Henkens, K. (2005). Couples' adjustment to retirement: A multi-actor panel study. *Journal of Gerontology: Social Sciences, 60B*, S11-S20.

W. T. Grant Consortium on the School-Based Promotion of Social Competence. (1992). Drug and alcohol prevention curricula. In J. D. Hawkins & R. F. Catalano (Eds.), *Communities that care: Action for drug abuse prevention* (pp.129-148). San Francisco, CA: Jossey-Bass.

Wang, M. (2007). Profiling retirees in the retirement transition and adjustment process: Examining the longitudinal change patterns of retirees' psychological well-being. *Journal of Applied Psychology, 92*, 455-474.

Wang, M., & Bodner, T. E. (2007). Growth mixture modeling: Identifying and predicting unobserved subpopulations with longitudinal data. *Organizational Research Methods, 10*, 635-656.

Wang, M., Henkens, K., & van Solinge, H. (2011). Retirement adjustment: A review of theoretical and empirical advancements. *American Psychologist, 66*(3), 204-213.

Wang, M., & Shultz, K. S. (2010). Employee retirement: A review and recommendations for future investigation. *Journal of Management, 36*, 172-206.

Watkins, D. C., Hunt, J. B., & Eisenberg, D. (2012). Increased demand for mental health services on college campuses: Perspectives from administrators. *Qualitative Social Work, 11*(3), 319-337.

Wood, M. (2012). The state of mental health on college campuses. *Inquiry, 17*(1), 5-15.

Wu, A. M. S., Tang, C. S. K., & Yan, E. C. W. (2005). Post-retirement voluntary work and psychological functioning among older Chinese in Hong Kong. *Journal of Cross-Cultural Gerontology, 20*, 27-4.

Zaff, J. F., Moore, K. A., Papillo, A. R., & Williams, S. (2003). Implications of extracurricular activity participation during adolescence on positive outcomes. *Journal of Adolescent Research, 18*, 599-630.

Zhan, Y., Wang, M., Liu, S., & Shultz, K. (2009). Bridge employment and retirees' health: A longitudinal investigation. *Journal of Occupational Health Psychology, 14*, 374-389.

EXERCISE

In: Positive Human Functioning ... Volume 2 ISBN: 978-1-62948-973-5
Editors: A. R. Gomes, R. Resende and A. Albuquerque © 2014 Nova Science Publishers, Inc.

Chapter 6

PREDICTING AND CHANGING EXERCISE BEHAVIOR: BRIDGING THE INFORMATION-INTENTION-BEHAVIOR GAP

James E. Maddux[1] and Kimberley A. Dawson[2]

[1] Department of Psychology & Center for the Advancement of Well-Being, George Mason University, Virginia, US

[2] Department of Kinesiology and Physical Education, Wilfrid Laurier University, Waterloo, Canada

ABSTRACT

The goal of this chapter is to provide a summary of theory and research on the *prediction* of exercise behavior and on the effectiveness of *interventions* designed to facilitate the initiation and maintenance of regular exercise. Information about the benefits of exercise easily leads to changes in intentions to exercise, but research has shown most people find it difficult to translate changes in intentions to changes in behavior, especially enduring changes in behavior. Special attention will be paid, therefore, to theory and research in bridging the information-intention-behavior gap. Toward this end, the chapter draws upon theory and research to offer a number of practical suggestions for changing and maintaining exercise behavior.

INTRODUCTION

Physical fitness (cardiopulmonary capacity, muscle strength and endurance, and flexibility) is one of the keys to a longer, healthier, happier life. Regular exercise is one of the most important contributors to physical fitness and to the prevention of a host of physical and psychological problems. The United States Centers for Disease Control and Prevention (2011) defines exercise as "physical activity that is planned, structured, repetitive, and purposive in the sense that the improvement or maintenance of one or more components of physical fitness is the objective."

Regular exercise has significant physical and psychological benefits. It reduces the risk of heart disease, colon cancer, Type 2 diabetes, osteoporosis, and hypertension (United States Department of Health and Human Services, 1996; Warburton, Nicol, and Bredin, 2006). It enhances weight control; maintenance of healthy bones, muscles and joints; physical strength and endurance United States Department of Health and Human Services (USDHHS), 1996; Warburton et al., 2006). It also can enhance self-esteem and feelings of subjective well-being and reduce depression, anxiety, and stress (Dishman and Duckworth, 1998; Tkachuk and Martin, 1999; Warburton et al., 2006). The World Health Organization (WHO) has also identified physical activity as a major contributor to overall physical health and to the prevention of numerous unhealthy conditions (see also Weinstein, this volume).

To accrue these benefits, the Unites States Department of Health and Human Services recommends a regimen of a half-hour of moderate exercise (e.g., walking) five times a week or 20 minutes of vigorous exercise (e.g., running) three times a week. These recommendations are similar to those of the American College of Sports Medicine (2011), which suggests 30 minutes of moderate intensity physical activity 5 days per week. The Canadian Society for Exercise Physiology (2011) offered more evidence-based physical activity guidelines for adults 18-64 suggesting that in order to achieve health benefits, adults should accumulate at least 150 minutes of moderate-to-vigorous intensity aerobic physical activity per week, in bouts of 10 minutes or more and to add muscle and bone strengthening activities using major muscle groups at least 2 days per week.

Despite the proven health benefits of regular physical activity mentioned above, only about 25% of adults in the United States exercise at the general frequency and intensity recommendations (Centers for Disease Control and Prevention, 2000; Nied and Franklin, 2002). In Canada, recent statistics based on the 2008 Physical Activity Monitor (Canadian Fitness and Lifestyle Institute, CFLRI: http://www.cflri.ca) suggest that only 49% of all Canadians (older than 20 years) are classified as at least moderately active and the majority of adults do not exercise sufficiently for health benefits to begin to accrue (Cameron, Wolfe, and Craig, 2007). Attrition rates (dropping out) from formal and informal exercise regimens average about 50% (Dishman, 1994). This statistic has remained constant over time.

The goal of this chapter is to provide a summary of theory and research on the prediction of exercise behavior and on the effectiveness of interventions designed to facilitate the initiation and maintenance of regular exercise. Special attention will be paid to the relationship between intentions to change exercise behaviour, which are relatively easy to influence, and actual changes in exercise behavior, which are much more difficult to influence.

PREDICTORS OF EXERCISE BEHAVIOR

Demographic Characteristics

Demographic data are not particularly good predictors of exercise behavior for either adults or children (Lee, 1993; Sallis, Prochaska, Taylor, Hill, and Geraci, 1999), although research has found some relationships between age and exercise. For example, beginning at around age six, physical activity generally declines with age (Lee, 1993; Malina, 1996;

Stephens, Jacobs, and White, 1985). At all ages, males are more physically active, on the average, than females (Stephens et al., 1985; USDHHS, 1996). Men are more likely than women to maintain changes in exercise following formal or structured interventions (Marcus et al., 2000). Men and women sometimes have different notions of what "exercise" means. For example, women are more likely than men to consider walking a form of exercise and to believe that it will enhance health (Lombard, Lombard, and Winett, 1995). Some evidence suggests that self-efficacy beliefs and planning are more important for women than for men in predicting exercise behavior (Hankonen, Pilvikki, Ghisletta, Renner, and Uutela, 2010). Single people of both genders are more active than are their married counterparts (Wankel, 1987).

Race and ethnicity are also associated with exercise. Among African American youth, about 15% are mostly inactive, compared to about 9% of Caucasian youth, and the differences between young African American and Caucasian girls is even greater (21% inactive versus 11%, respectively) (USDHHS, 1996). This difference extends to adults. In the U.S., sedentary behavior is more common among African American adults (38%) than among Latino adults (35%) and Caucasian adults (27%) (Centers for Disease Control and Prevention, 2009). Income and education levels also appear to be related to physical activity patterns. Low income groups participate in less physical activity than the overall population (Lox, Martin Ginis, and Petruzzello, 2010). The higher an individual's level of education, the more likely that individual is to engage in regular physical activity (Lox et al., 2010). Poorer people (incomes < $10,000) are less active than are wealthier people (income > $50,000) (41.5% inactive and 17.8% inactive, respectively) (USDHHS, 1996).

According to the Kids CANPLAY! 2011 bulletin (CFLRI: http:// www.cflri.ca), Canadian children demonstrate the same activity trends as adults. Boys take more daily steps, on average, than girls do and the number of steps taken decrease with age. Gender differences exist at every age group with boys and girls equally decreasing their daily steps over time. Children from University educated parents and living in the highest income households (>$100,000.00 per year) also take more daily steps on average than those from households with lower education and incomes. One can assume that these demographic patterns are similar to those of other industrialized nations, with physical activity decreasing with age throughout the lifespan.

Personality Traits

The search for personality traits that predict health behavior in general and exercise in particular has not uncovered much useful information (e.g., Willis and Campbell, 1992). The personality trait that has been investigated the most is *locus-of-control*—the general belief that one's behavior has an impact on one's environment. The more specific notion of *health locus-of-control* (the one's behavior can have an impact on one's health) also has received considerable attention. Research suggests, however, that measures of general locus-of-control and health locus-of-control are not good predictors of who will or will not exercise (Biddle, 1999; Sallis and Owen, 1999). In addition, exercise behavior has been found to be positively associated with extraversion and emotional intelligence and negatively associated with neuroticism (Saklofske, Austin, and Rohr, 2006). Gender does not appear to influence the relationship between personality and exercise (Lochbaum, Rhodes, Stevenson, Surles, Stevens, and Wang, 2010).

People who score higher on measures of *optimism* exercise more than those scoring lower (Kavussanu and McAuley, 1995) and generally tend to report better overall health-related quality of life (e.g., Peterson et al., 2008). What is not clear, however, is whether being more optimistic leads one to exercise more or whether exercise makes one more optimistic. People who are more optimistic are probably more likely to believe that exercise will produce desirable benefits (positive outcome expectancies), that they can perform exercise behaviors (positive self-efficacy expectancies), and that they can overcome the barriers to exercising that are common in daily life (also an aspect of self-efficacy), notions that will be discussed further in a later section of this chapter. These exercising optimists then reap the additional psychological and emotional benefit of their exercise, which could lead to greater optimism, and which then leads to greater activity, as suggested by the *broaden-and-build* theory of emotion (Frederickson, 2001).

Social and Interpersonal Influences

The support of important others in a person's life can influence exercise behavior (e.g., Fraser and Rodgers, 2012). Almost two-thirds of adults who exercise regularly do so with other people (Stephens and Craig, 1990), and the exercise behavior of men, women, and children is strongly influenced by the reactions of other people (Carron, Hausenblas, and Mack, 1996; Oka, King, and Young, 1995; Sallis, Prochaska, Taylor, Hill, and Geraci, 1999; Tucker and Mueller, 2000). Spouses can encourage exercise by modeling the behavior, discussing health-related issues, and providing emotional support (Tucker and Mueller, 2000). Providing reassurances of worth, attachment, and guidance can enhance attendance at exercise classes (Duncan, McAuley, Stoolmiller, and Duncan, 1993). For some people, the support provided by fitness clubs members and staff is more important than support from family and friends (DuCharme, Widmeyer, Dorsch, and Hoar, 1996). In exercise groups, the cohesion of the group is an important predictor of adherence (King, Taylor, Haskell, and DeBusk, 1990), especially in the early phases of the group. The support of peers can also be important in encouraging exercise among high school students (Bunke, Apitzch, and Baeckstroem, 2013) and college students (Gruber, 2008).

Social support is effective because other people influence our beliefs about cognitive factors such self-efficacy beliefs (Carron, Hausenblas, and Mack, 1996; Duncan and McAuley, 1993). In addition, the desire for the approval of important others can influence the motivation to adhere to exercise regimens, as suggested in the theory of reasoned action/planned behavior (to be discussed in a later section of this chapter). Many people exercise because it offers an opportunity to be with other people. As noted previously, the social incentives for exercising can increase in importance over time.

Social support is also affected by the *type* of exercise interventions. Tracey, Dawson, and Berry (2009) compared two physical activity interventions: traditional group-based and internet-based. Individuals in the group intervention reported liking both the social aspects of the group and the accountability. The also reported liking the information that was presented and believed that it was relevant to them. The internet based group, however, reported that they missed the social contact and that the information provided on the website was not new or relevant to their specific needs. The authors concluded that only the traditional group-based intervention contained the social support necessary for successful long-term exercise behavior change.

While social support is generally viewed as a positive influence on exercise participation, it can, at times, have a detrimental affect. When individuals believe that significant others are trying to control or manipulate them by encouraging them to exercise, they may engage in behavioral reactance and actually exercise less (Lewis and Rook, 1999; Lox et al, 2010). In order for social support to facilitate exercise behavior, the support provided must be congruent in both type and amount with the support desired and required. The exerciser must also perceive the support as helpful, not controlling, in order for the support to be effective in motivating behavior change. While a spouse may *think* that he or she is being supportive by buying a gym a membership for his or her partner, the partner may *perceive* that this is an attempt to control his or her free time. Anecdotal evidence also suggests that a spouse may view this as criticism or even an insult. As a result, the partner may refrain from using the gym membership in order to reestablish a sense of personal control through noncompliance. As with many other health behaviors, social support for exercise must be provided in moderation to be effective. Both too little and too much can be detrimental for sustained exercise change.

Program Characteristics

Exercise behavior can be influenced by *type* of program and by the *match* between person and type of exercise program. Adherence is likely to be better across all types of programs if people's preferences for one type over another are taken into account, particularly in the initial stages of a program (King et al., 1997). Exercising in a true group is more effective than a standard exercise class (Burke, Carron, Eys, Ntoumanis, and Estabrooks, 2006). Exercising at home with contact from a researcher or health-care professional is as effective as exercising in a standard group or class (Burke et al., 2006). Exercising at home with contact is more effective than exercising at home without contact (Burke et al., 2006).

Long-term adherence (two years) among both men and women is better for *supervised home-based programs* than for group programs (King, Haskell, Young, Oka, and Stefanick, 1995; King, Kiernan, Oman, Kraemer, Hull, and Ahn, 1997). Home-based programs have been shown to be more effective in producing long-term adherence than supervised programs that take place outside the home (Ashworth, Chad, Harrison, Reeder, and Marshall, 2005; Garcia and King, 1991). In addition, interventions may be more effective if they are targeted for an individual's readiness for change and his or her stage in the behavior-change process (e.g., contemplating change, intending to initiate change) (Lippke, Schwarzer, Zieglemann, Scholz, and Schulz, 2010).

The relationship between intensity and adherence seems influenced by frequency. Some studies have found greater maintenance at two years for a high-intensity home-based program than for a low-intensity home-based program, perhaps because the high-intensity regimen required a lower frequency than the low-intensity program (King et al., 1995).

The *accessibility* of the location where exercise occurs (e.g., a gym or health club) and its distance from home or work can influence adherence; more accessible and closer locations produce greater adherence rates (Cox, 1984; Reed and Phillips, 2005; Wankel, 1985).

Likewise, *physical characteristics* of an exercise facility such as layout, size, and age influence attendance (Willis and Campbell, 1992). Finally, simple reminders or *prompts* (e.g., weekly phone calls, mailings) are effective in increasing and maintaining adherence to exercise regimens (e.g., Burke et al., 2006, King et al., 1990; Lombard et al., 1995).

Situational Cues

Situational cues influence behavior in two ways. First, a situation may contain action cues such that a behavior performed frequently in that situation may eventually come to be automatically triggered in that situation without the individual's intention or awareness. We call such behaviors habits (Orbell and Verplanken, 2010). For example, someone might automatically lock the doors and fasten the seatbelt when getting into the driver's side of his or her own automobile but not when getting into the backseat of a taxi. Second, for other behaviors, including most health behaviors, certain situations may contain decision cues that elicit the cognitive factors involved in the formation of intentions and action plans (Oettingen and Gollwitzer, 2010). For example, good weather or the sight of one's running shoes or bicycle may initiate a process of deciding whether or not to go for a run or a ride. Seeing a television commercial for athletic gear or a health club may be a cue for deciding whether or not to finally join a gym.

Life Events

The maintenance of an exercise regimen can be derailed by *life events* both minor and major. Minor *daily hassles* (e.g., hurrying to meet a deadline at work, too many responsibilities) can disrupt the performance of planned exercise, reduce the time spent exercising, and diminish self-efficacy for and satisfaction with exercise (Stetson, Rahn, Dubbert, Wilner, and Mercury, 1997). *Major life events* such as change in employment status and change in residence can significantly disrupt maintenance of exercise regimens (Allender, Hutchinson, and Foster, 2008; Oman and King, 2000). Two major life events are usually insufficient to cause major disruption of an exercise regimen, but three or more events usually will do the trick (Oman and King, 2000).

Cognitive Variables

Cognitions are what people think and believe. The vast majority of research on the cognitive predictors of exercise (and health behavior more generally) has been based on one or more of the various social cognitive theories such as protection motivation theory, the health belief model, self-efficacy theory, the theories of reasoned action and planned behavior, and stages of change theories such as the transtheoretical model (Dawson, Robertson-Wilson, and Martin Ginis, 2011) and the health adoption process approach (Maddux, 1993, 2007; Schwarzer, 2008). The most important assumption of these models is that situational events, environmental events, cognition, emotion, and behavior are mutually interacting influences and that a complete understanding of human behavior in any situation requires an understanding of all of these sources of influences and how they interact (Bandura, 1997; Maddux, 2010). A second crucial assumption is that people engage in self-regulation (intentional control over one's own behavior) by envisioning goals and by using these goals to create incentives and plans that motivate and guide their behavior (Bandura, 2001; Maddux, 2009). These models share several basic conceptual building blocks, including (1) goals, (2) plans, (3) behavior-outcome expectancies, (4) outcome value, (5) self-efficacy expectancies, and (6) behavioral intentions.

A goal is what a person would like to accomplish or achieve. Goals are not mystical or magical. Setting a goal will not automatically lead to goal attainment. Instead, in order for goals to be effective and change behavior, they must be mechanistic. According to Locke and Latham (2002), effective goals change behavior in four ways. First, they motivate individuals to search for effective behavioral strategies required to reach the goal. Second, they remind individuals to exert effort in attempting goal attainment. Third, they motivate individuals to persist when they are challenged with obstacles. Finally, goals help individuals keep their focus and attention on the goal when rival options present themselves. Goals are an effective motivational piece of the exercise behavior change journey (Dawson and Brawley, 2000).

A plan is the person's strategy for achieving the goal. Action plans are a key element of engaging in a regular exercise program. Having a goal provides the impetus for establishing clear and reliable behavioral plans. Setting a target alone will not be productive, unless the individual knows what the behaviors are that are required to meet that goal. For example, a goal of losing five pounds will never come to fruition if the individual does not know that he or she must increase activity and decrease caloric consumption in order to reach it. Effective behavioral planning involves finding successful actions for the short term as well as the long term by anticipating difficult or potentially problematic situations. Similar to sports, with voluntary exercise, the best offense is often the best defense. By anticipating barriers to exercising and planning on how to alleviate them, challenges will be more easily averted or overcome when they present themselves.

A behavior-outcome expectancy is a belief about the contingency between a specific behavior and a specific outcome (result, consequence) or set of outcomes (Maddux, 1999). Much of people's plans consist of such expectancies. Behavior-outcome expectancies are good predictors of exercise behavior (Courneya, 1995; Lee, 1993). People are likely to drop out of exercise programs if they have unrealistic expectations about the immediacy of its benefits (Desharnais, Bouillon, and Godin, 1986). People's expectations that they will encounter practical barriers to regular exercise also predict their level of physical activity (Lee, 1993). Research also suggests an important distinction between exercise-related affective (emotions) outcome expectancies, and health-related outcome expectancies (Gellert, Ziegelmann, and Schwarzer, 2012).

Outcome value is the importance attached to specific outcomes in specific situations (Maddux, 1999). An outcome can be valued because a person wishes to attain it (e.g., a trimmer physique, better health) or because the person wishes to avoid it (e.g., cancer, obesity). The importance of outcome value in health-related behavior has been demonstrated by a considerable body of research (e.g., Rogers and Prentice-Dunn, 1997; Strecher, Champion, and Rosenstock, 1997). The values of outcomes are not static but can change over time. For example, people often begin exercise programs for the expected physical health and appearance benefits, but over time mood enhancement and social benefits become increasingly important incentives (Hsiao and Thayer, 1997).

A self-efficacy expectancy or belief is a judgment concerning one's ability to execute a behavior or course of action. Self-efficacy beliefs are important because they influence the goals people set, their persistence in pursuing their goals, and their emotional reactions to perceived success and failure (Bandura, 1997). Self-efficacy for performing specific exercise behaviors, scheduling exercise sessions, and overcoming barriers to exercising are all good predictors of exercise (Courneya, 1995; Cramp and Brawley, 2006; Dawson and Brawley, 2000; Dawson, Brawley, and Maddux, 2000; Dawson, Tracey, and Berry, 2008; Hu, Motl, McAuley, and Konopack, 2007; McAuley and Courneya, 1993). Self-efficacy for recovery from setbacks in maintaining an exercise regimen seems to be particularly important predicting exercise behavior (Lusczcynska, Mazurkiewicz, Ziegelmann, and Schwarzer, 2007). In addition, people who believe that physical ability can be enhanced through practice are less likely to experience negative affect and are more likely to persist in the face of difficulty than those who believe that physical ability is an immutable characteristic (Kasimatis, Miller, and Marcussen, 1996).

A behavioral intention is what one says one will do. An behavioral intention is not a goal, although one can intend to attain a goal. Instead, behavioral intentions are concerned with the behaviors one might engage in to attain a goal (Maddux, 1999). Of particular importance are implementation intentions or intentions to perform specific behaviors in specific situations because they increase the probability that the person will perform a goal-related behavior when provided the opportunity to do so (Oettingen and Gollwitzer, 2010; Prestwick, Lawton, Conner, 2003). Because this chapter is concerned with bridging the gap between behavioral intentions and actual behavior, behavioral intentions will be discussed in greater detail.

THEORIES INVOLVING BEHAVIORAL INTENTIONS

Theory of Reasoned Action and Planned Behavior

The notion of behavioral intentions was first featured prominently in the theory of reasoned action (Fishbein and Ajzen, 1975) and its revision, the theory of planned behavior (Ajzen, 1985). These theories assume that people make rational decisions about their behavior based on their beliefs about the behavior and its consequences. These beliefs include *attitudes* toward the behavior, which consist of beliefs about expected consequences (outcome expectancies) and the importance of those consequences (outcome value or valence). They also include the person's perceptions of *social norms* regarding the behavior—beliefs that important others believe that the person should or should not perform the behavior and the person's motivation to comply with these others—that is, the person's expectations regarding the possible reactions of other people and the important placed on those reactions. Both attitudes and perceived social norms influence the person's *intentions* to perform the behavior, which are viewed as the most proximal influences over behavior.

The theory of planned behavior builds on the theory of reasoned action by proposing that predictions of intentions and behavior must include an assessment of the person's *perceived control* over the behavior—a concept almost identical to the notion of *self-efficacy* beliefs in that both involve one's beliefs that one has the resources and opportunities to execute the behavior in question.

Protection Motivation Theory

Protection motivation theory (PMT) was developed originally to explain inconsistencies in the research on fear appeals and attitude change (Rogers, 1975) but since has been employed primarily as a model for health-related decision making and behavior change. In PMT, decisions to engage (or not engage) in health-related behaviors are influenced by two primary cognitive processes. *Threat appraisal* is an evaluation of the factors that influence the likelihood of engaging in an unhealthy behavior and consists of two components: *perceived vulnerability*—an estimation of the likelihood of harm should one continue engaging in the unhealthy behavior, and *perceived severity*—an estimation of the magnitude of harm. *Coping appraisal* is an evaluation of the factors influencing the likelihood of engaging in a preventive response (healthy behavior) and also consists of two components: *response efficacy*—an estimation of the likelihood that the proposed preventive behavior will be effective, and *self-efficacy*, the belief in one's ability to implement the preventive behavior or coping strategy (Maddux and Rogers, 1983).

Threat appraisal and coping appraisal directly influence *intentions* to give up the unhealthy behavior and adopt the healthy behavior.

Health Action Process Approach

The basic problem with protection motivation theory and the theory of planned behavior (and other similar theories) is that research continues to show that these theories are good predictors of exercise intentions but relatively weak predictors of exercise behavior (e.g., Hobbs, Dixon, Johnston, and Howie, 2013; Plotnikoff, Lubans, Trinh, and Craig, 2011; Vallance, Lavalee, Culos-Reed, and Trudeau, 2012). The health action process approach (HAPA) (Lippke and Plotnikoff, 2013; Schwarzer, 2008) was developed specifically to address this "behavior-intention gap". The HAPA incorporates the linear or continuous variables found in the theory of reasoned action/planned behavior, protection motivation theory, and other theories not reviewed here (e.g., risk perceptions, outcome expectancies, self-efficacy beliefs, behavioral intentions) into a type of stage model, with the "stages" conceptualized more accurately as qualitatively different phases or mindsets (i.e., set of cognitions or beliefs). The HAPA views health behavior change as consisting of two major stages or mindsets: (1) a preintentional motivational stage in which the individual (referred to as a "preintender") sets goals and forms behavioral intentions, and (2) a postintentional volitional stage in which the individual eventually engages in actual attempts at behavior change. In this second stage, individuals can be divided further into two groups (or stages): (1) individuals who have not yet translated their intentions and goals into action ("intenders"), and (2) those who have made attempts at behavior change ("actors").

As noted previously, one of the major problems with most theories of health-related behavior change is their failure to predict or explain how behavioral intentions become translated in actual behavior and how the individual copes with barriers and setbacks during attempts to change behavior. These models also do not take into account the changes in the influence of their major components, such as perceptions of risk, severity of expected harm, goals, intentions, and self-efficacy beliefs. The HAPA attempts to bridge the intention-behavior gap by proposing that in the postintentional stage, planning (also referred as at implementation intentions; Gollwitzer, 1999) mediates the transition from intending to acting - a transition that has also been referred to as *action control* (de Bruijn, Verkooijen, de Vries, and van den Putte, 2012).

Planning (implementation intentions) consists of intentions to engage in specific behavior at specific times, in specific places, and under specific conditions (e.g., "When I am at a party and someone offers me a cigarette, I will politely say 'No thank you, I am trying to quit' and eat a carrot instead."). This type of situation-specific planning leads to greater automaticity of behavior in the presence of situational cues (Rhodes, Fiala, and Nasuti, 2012). Planning is divided into two types: *action planning* (plans for implementing the desired behavior change—when, where, and how to act) and *coping planning* (plans for dealing with barriers and setbacks). Research suggests that having both an action plan and a coping plan is better than having just one or the other and that having several plans is better than just having one (Wiedemann, Lippke, Reuter, Ziegelmann, and Schulz, 2010). Research also suggests that planning can be enhanced through prompts (reminders) and instructions (Evers, Klusmann, Schwarzer, and Heuser, 2011; Evers, Klusmann, Ziegelmann, Schwarzer, and Heuser, 2012; Fleig, Lippke, Pomp, and Schwarzer, 2011). Some evidence suggests that planning is more important for women than for men in predicting exercise behavior (Hankonen et al., 2010).

Research has found support for the model's distinction between the preintentional motivational stage and the postintentional volitional stage by revealing differences between these stages on measures of risk perception, outcome expectancies, self-efficacy beliefs, goals, and action planning. More specifically, as predicted by the model, research has found that intenders and actors differ on measures of self-efficacy, goals, and action planning but not on measures of risk perception and outcome expectancies (Lippke and Plotnikoff, 2013). Research also supports the distinction between types of self-efficacy beliefs at different stages, including task self-efficacy, coping self-efficacy, and recovery self-efficacy (Lippke and Plotnikoff, 2013; Schwarzer, 2008). Finally, research has supported the importance of the distinction between action planning, which seems most important at the adoption stage, and coping planning (or barrier management), which seems most important in the maintenance stage (Fuchs, Seelig, Goehner, Burton, and Brown, 2012).

The relation between planning and behavior is mediated and moderated by several other variables. For example, people whose motivations to exercise are autonomous—that is, more *intrinsic* (motivated by the satisfaction derived from engaging in the behavior itself rather than *extrinsic* (motivated by external rewards) are more likely to translate intentions into behaviors (Cao, Lippke, and Wei, 2011; Jackson, Whipp, Chua, Dimmock, and Hagger, 2013). The greater a person's sense of identity as an exercise (e.g., being an exercise is consistent with self-concept), the more like the person is to make the transition from intentions to behavior (de Bruijn et al., 2012). People who have experience with planning their activities in other domains are more likely to have good planning skills, and these planning experiences predict the ability to plan exercise activities. Fortunately, planning skills can be easily taught (Cao, Schuez, Xie, and Lippke, 2013). In addition, planning seems to be effective even when people cannot later recall the plans that they had developed (Wiedemann, Lippke, and Schwarzer, 2011).

Planning seems to be especially important for people with a more limited future time perspective—for example, older adults who realistically view their futures as more limited than do younger adults. The more limited a person's future time perspective (typically related to chronlogical age), the less likely that person is to make the transition from intentions to behavior (Hall, Fong, and Cheng, 2012) and the more likely that person is to benefit from planning (Gellert, Zigelmann, Lippke, and Schwarzer, 2012).

Self-efficacy appears to be essential for planning to effectively mediate the relation between intentions and behavior (Koring, Richert, Parschau, Lippke, and Schwarzer, 2012; Luszczynzka, Schwarzer, Lippke, and Mazurkiewicz, 2011). The importance of self-efficacy may explain why depression interferes with the effectiveness of interventions designed to enhance self-regulation skills (Pomp, Fleig, Schwarzer, and Lippke, 2013).

The results of research on the HAPA are generally consistent with others studies concerned with stages of behavior change (e.g., Dishman and Sallis, 1994, Prochaska and Prochaska, 2010; Rothman, 2000), although the HAPA deals in greater detail with the relation between intention and behavior and the importance of planning in mediating this relation. For example, research suggests that self-efficacy beliefs may be more important predictors of behavior for beginning exercisers than for experienced or habitual exercisers (Dawson and Brawley, 2000). Dawson et al. (2008) used a stage-matched approach in their comparison of a traditional cognitive-behavioral group based intervention with an internet intervention in a workplace. Results demonstrated that more than a statistically expected number of participants in the preparation stage were found in both intervention groups. More individuals in the maintenance stages of exercise selected the internet-based intervention over the group-based intervention. This study demonstrates how individuals in different stages differ in their preferences for intervention delivery modes (Dawson et al., 2011).

Bridging the Information-Intention-Behavior Gap

Knowing what predicts exercise behavior is useful only if this knowledge can be used to design interventions to increase the likelihood that people will initiate and maintain regular exercise regimens. Genetically endowed biological capacities, personality traits, gender, age, ethnicity, income, and marital status are resistant to change, to say the least. For this reason, most of the research on interventions to has focused on what can be changed—*cognitive factors* and *program factors*. Unfortunately, intervention research has not been as plentiful or fruitful as the research on prediction. Many of these interventions have produced robust changes in cognitions (e.g., expected benefits, self-efficacy) but fewer have produced significant changes in behavior (Baranowski, Anderson, and Carmack, 1998; Dawson et al., 2011).

Simply providing information about the benefits of exercise, although important in early stages of changes (as in the HAPA preintention motivational stage), rarely is sufficient to produce enduring behavior change. Even constructing persuasive communications based on exercise information relevant to the participants does not always increase physical activity participation (Chatzisarantis and Hagger, 2005). However, providing additional information on how to change behavior more systematically (e.g., instructions on self-monitoring, planning, scheduling of activities) may motivate some people to initiate behavior change. Such people, however, are likely to be those who already are good self-regulators in other areas of their lives. In addition, encouraging people to exercise with a partner or in a group will probably get some people off the sofa and into the gym or onto the jogging trail. The more reluctant among the sedentary (probably the majority), however, are not likely to be motivated into action by either of these strategies. In addition, research suggests that those who begin are likely to flounder and quit within a few months.

What is most likely to work is a structured, multiple-component intervention that employs a variety of strategies.

Information

A necessary but certainly not sufficient condition for encouraging exercise behavior is providing people with information about the perils of a sedentary lifestyle, the benefits of a more active lifestyle, and what they need to do to become more active in a way that will produce benefits to their health. People must be informed about the numerous physical and psychological benefits of exercise and the perils of a sedentary lifestyle. This information usually takes the form of behavior-outcomes expectancies and outcome values, which are components found in all the theories of health behavior. Information about the dangers of inactivity should be designed to raise concern and motivation but not to instill too much fear because doing so may lead to avoidance rather than constructive action (Witte and Allen, 2000). It is the value aspect of the information that is crucial for behavior change. Information targeting children and youth should include the social benefits of exercise rather than the health outcomes because the most important health outcomes are in the future. Conversely, identifying the health benefits of exercise for older adults could be extremely important.

In most of the economically developed world, people are already well aware that regular exercise is good for them, yet relatively few engage in it. Simply repeating such information is unlikely to have much of an impact on most sedentary people. Information is a necessary first step, but not the only step, required for behavioral change. As multiple public health initiatives have discovered, education and information are not enough to evoke large scale population changes. The Canadian Participation media campaigns have attempted to change public exercise rates, however, Canadians still remain largely sedentary despite this effort.

Setting Goals

Effective behavior change and maintenance of that change (i.e., self-regulation) requires clear and specific goals. Therefore, people must decide which of the many benefits of exercise are most important to them: making new friends; enhancing health and athletic prowess; increasing physical attractiveness; recovering from an illness or injury; preventing disease and disability; or managing stress, anxiety, or depression. Setting clear and specific goals and sub-goals makes it easier for people to gather information about their progress (feedback) and to modify their behavior in a way that facilitates progress toward the goal. It may also be helpful to persuade people that exercise can be enjoyable so that intrinsic motivations and goals are added to the mix in addition to more extrinsic motivations and goals.

Developing Intrinsic Exercise Goals (Autonomous Motivation)

Although most sedentary people are likely to begin exercising because of the expected health benefits (extrinsic motivation), they are more likely to successfully maintain those behavioral changes if they begin to view exercise as rewarding in and of itself, apart from the expected health benefits.

Developing an "Exerciser" Identity

Intentionally beginning to view oneself as "a person who exercises" may increase the probability that exercise behavior will be maintained, possibly because not exercising eventually becomes incongruent with one's new identity as an exerciser.

Developing Action Plans

People must develop a action plan that includes at least the following components.

- A breakdown of long-term goals into manageable *short-term goals. Graded mastery experiences* that increase in frequency, duration, and/or intensity will help people experience initial success, which leads to greater self-efficacy, which in turn encourages people to set slightly higher goals and to persevere toward them.
- The identification of what behaviors must to be performed and in what situations (where and when) they should be performed. This specificity leads to the development of *implementation intentions* (intentions to perform specific behaviors in specific situations), which increase the probability that the person will engage in goal-directed behavior when given the opportunity to do so.
- Time-management. Deliberately scheduling exercise periods into one's weeks and days is more effective than simply hoping to "get around to it" when one has taken care of other responsibilities. The benefits of scheduling derive partly from the influence of implementation intentions. Time management is particularly important at the beginning of an exercise program when many people have difficulty envisioning the possibility of making time in their busy schedules for exercise.
- Development of Plan A, B, and C. An effective Plan A (action plan) is based on developing strategies for maintaining a regular exercise program under normal life situations. An effective Plan B (coping plan) is determined in advance of times when schedule change and anticipated barriers occur. Both Plans A and B are established in advance of the exercise program. A Plan C should be implemented at times when it is necessary to salvage any semblance of an exercise program during unforeseen or unpredictable situations. For example, Plan A is used to regulate exercise during a normal work week. Plan B is utilized to manage exercise when a schedule may change during the week when a major presentation is due and requires more time commitment. Plan C is used in the overseen circumstances of being housebound to attend to a sick child. Plan C involves adjusting to the immediate circumstances and

using the resources at hand such running up and down stairs for the day. A Plan C is developed when some exercise is better than no exercise at all.

Developing Coping Plans

People need to be assisted in developing plans for dealing with the barriers and setbacks that are inevitable in attempting long-term change in physical activity. These plans should include:

- Anticipating potential *barriers* to exercise—that is, situations and events likely to result in *relapse* (e.g., fatigue, emotional distress, daily hassles, major life events, working late, inclement weather, travelling) and a *strategy* for overcoming each of these barriers.
- Novice exercisers should remind themselves continually that success is not linear, that setbacks and relapses are a normal part of process, and that relapses should be viewed not as failures but as opportunities to exercise their self-regulatory abilities. Acknowledging the inevitability of relapses will increase the probability that the person will recover from the relapse and get back to his or her routine rather than view the relapse as an indication of personal failure or physical incapability.

Using Physical Activity Contracts and Behavioral Monitoring

Contracts enhance an individual's commitment and motivation to attain the exercise goal (Dawson et al., 2011). The contract identifies the desired exercise goal and details about consequences (e.g., rewards) for attaining the goal (Berger, Pargman, and Weinberg, 2002). Cress and colleagues (2005) concluded that physical activity contracts are extremely effective among older adults. Keeping track of the exercise behavior and the accompanying emotions and cognitions (behavior monitoring) can also be effective (Buckworth and Dishman, 2002).

Choosing the Right Exercise Program

A careful match of the exercise regimen with the person's needs, preferences, and lifestyle probably will enhance adherence. Various options include structured programs (e.g., classes at a gym, church, or community center), unstructured solo programs (e.g., walking or running alone), team sports (e.g., basketball and soccer leagues), and informal group activities (e.g., running clubs). In addition, for some people the demands of work and family may require a more flexible program than for others. People who are easily bored with repetitive activity may be better suited for team sports than for solo exercising or a regularly scheduled aerobics class. Some people enjoy exercising alone (which gives them control over what, when, and how long), while others prefer the social benefits of a small group. Gender differences should be considered. As noted previously, men are less likely than women to view walking as "exercise" and may fare better in an activity that is sport-related. A Physical Activity Counselor (PAC), who is a trained member of the health care team and able to prescribe more individually based exercise programs based on principles of behavior modification, was found to improve exercise activity (Blanchard et al., 2007). Individual needs assessments and realistic exercise prescription plans will yield the best results.

Engaging Social Support

Research on the social norms component of the theory of reason action/planned behavior indicates that other people are important in encouraging the initiation and maintenance in changes in attitudes and behavior. Engaging social support should include:

- Harnessing the assistance and *support* of friends, family, fellow exerciser, or a trainer. The support of important others should not be assumed; it should be arranged. The novice exerciser should tell other people what he/she is trying to accomplish and then should tell them how they can be supportive.
- Getting regular *feedback* on progress from a friend or family member (if an informal program) or trainer or group leader (if a formal program). Goals are ineffective without feedback. Positive feedback about performance can enhance self-efficacy, which can in turn increase positive effect and decrease negative affect during exercise, especially in the early stages of exercise adoption. This may, in turn, result in lower attrition and fewer missed exercise sessions.

Arranging Situational Decision Cues

As noted previously, exercise is not likely to become a habit that is automatically triggered by situational cues. Cognitions about exercise, however, can be triggered by situational cues, and one is more likely to exercise if one is thinking about it than if one is not. For this reason, people can arrange for situational cues that trigger thoughts about exercising, such as leaving one's exercise equipment and exercise clothing where they can be seen and not avoided, posting reminder notes, and sending oneself email or voice mail *prompts* (reminders).

Conclusion

Volitional exercise change is difficult for most individuals. While large scale health promotional campaigns geared toward other negative behaviors such as smoking and driving while intoxicated have been successful in changing both public awareness and engagement in these activities, these same large-based campaigns have been less successful when geared toward physical activity. Most exercise change occurs as a result of a forced change when loss of health is a reality. Although smoking is clearly viewed by the vast majority of people as harmful, not exercising is often viewed as neutral or non-harmful. It is important, therefore, that people come to understand that not engaging in physical activity is also detrimental to health because of the long-term negative affects of sedentariness on health.

While information alone is not enough, cognitive-behavioral interventions used in conjunction with this message may begin to shift behavior to a more active lifestyle. *Exercise is Medicine* (2012) is an initiative geared toward having all health care professionals design treatment plans as an integral part in the prevention and treatment of wellness. Physical inactivity is a major public health concern for all industrialized countries. Adopting physical activity assessment as a standard protocol in medical offices throughout the nation will significantly contribute to awareness of sedentary lifestyles. Again, increases in knowledge will have to be accompanied by individualized exercise behavioral plans to be effective.

The goal of much research on exercise has been to encourage everyone to exercise at the USDHHS recommended levels of intensity and frequency, as noted at the beginning of this entry. Research on attrition, however, suggests that this goal is unrealistic. Most people simply will not maintain exercise regimens at those recommended levels, and if people believe that those levels, which are difficult for most people to achieve, are necessary to reap meaningful health benefits, they are likely give up and return to doing nothing at all. Fortunately, compliance with USDHHS recommendations may be viewed in graduated steps, rather than in all or nothing terms. For example, evidence suggests that some of the traditional and accepted notions about the amount and frequency of exercise that is necessary to accrue health benefits may be inaccurate. Recent research suggests, for example, that even the smallest increases in exercise (e.g., brief walks scattered throughout the day) will result in some improvements in health (Canadian Society for Exercise Physiology, 2011). In addition, three periods of exercise of ten minutes each may be as effective as a single 30-minute episode (Haskell et al., 2007). Even if further research does indeed indicate that we have been asking people to do not just more than they are willing to do, but also more than they need to do, then what we have learned so far about promoting adherence to exercise regimens will nonetheless prove valuable.

Therefore, research on exercise motivation and adherence should focus less on how to get people to adhere to USDHHS standards as such and more on how to encourage people to make small changes in exercise behavior toward those standards based on more realistic expectations derived from each individual's goals, abilities, and limitations. The probability of enhancing physical fitness in the general population will be increased with well-planned and carefully executed interventions to encourage the initiation and maintenance of regular exercise regimens that take into consideration individual differences in ability, personal preferences, and lifestyle. Program planners (including researchers and healthcare professionals) need to make sure that they are trying to get people do to what really works and that they are not asking people to do more than they really need to do to attain their *own* desired level of fitness and meet their *own* goals. Most important, people cannot be simply provided with information and instructions and left to their own devices to implement recommendations. They need direct and specific instructions on how to translate good intentions into behavior change, primarily through direct and specific assistance in developing details plans of action and details plans for coping with barriers and setback. Doing so will increase the likelihood that sedentary people will make at least some modest changes and maintain them over time. Not everyone can (or even wants to) become an athlete, but everyone can improve his or her level of activity sufficient for increasing the length and quality of life.

Finally, ideas for changing exercise behavior can be found in research on a variety of health-related behaviors. From the standpoint of theory, the health-related behaviors that have received the most attention from researchers—exercise, smoking, alcohol abuse, diet, compliance with medical regimens, wearing seatbelts, safer sex practices, among others—are more similar than different. For example, viewed strictly through the lens of social-cognitive theories, the behaviors that lead to HIV infection are more similar to than different from the behaviors that contribute to the development of other health problems that have a largely behavioral genesis, such as smoking, alcohol abuse, over-eating, and chronic sedentariness. In each of these examples, the behaviors one must engage in are quite simple motorically (e.g., putting on a condom or putting out a cigarette). At the same time, however, these behaviors are associated with powerful human urges and powerful pleasures that are not easily resisted, especially when one is in a situation where these urges and pleasures are salient. Sexual drives are powerful indeed, but so are hunger, thirst, nicotine cravings, and the desire to avoid physical pain and discomfort.

These behaviors also share obstacles to change. The major obstacle to changing from an unhealthy behavior to a healthy behavior is the conflict between proximal (immediate) and distal (future) consequences and the power that proximal consequences exert over behavior. Most unhealthy behaviors are unhealthy only in the long run (after many repetitions) but are immediately pleasurable and gratifying. Likewise, changing from unhealthy to healthy behavior (e.g., getting up off the sofa and doing push-ups, pushing aside the mashed potatoes and eating the broccoli instead) almost always results in initial discomfort, pain, or deprivation. This conflict makes it difficult for people to put on condoms, put down cigarettes, eat fewer potatoes, eat more broccoli, and get up and do push-ups or go for a brisk walk. For these reasons, what research tells us how to discourage one unhealthy behaviors can likely tell us how to discourage others, and what research tell us about how to encourage one healthy behavior can likely tell us how to discourage others.

REFERENCES

Ajzen, I. (1985). From intentions to actions: A theory of planned behavior. In J. Kuhl and J. Beckman (Eds.), *Action-control: From cognition to behavior* (pp. 11-39). Heidelberg: Springer.

Allender, S., Hutchinson, L., and Foster, C. (2008). Life-change events and participation in physical activity: A systematic review. *Health Promotion International, 23,* 160-172.

American College of Sports Medicine. (2011). *Quantity and quality of exercise for developing and maintaining cardiorespiratory, musculoskeletal, and neuromotor fitness in relatively healthy adults: Guidance for prescribing exercise.* Retrieved September 6, 2011 from http://www.acsm.org/access-public-information/position-stands/position-stands/lists/position-stands/quantity-and-quality-of-exercise-for-developing-and-maintaining-cardiorespiratory-musculoskeletal-and-neuromotor-fitness-in-apparently-healthy-adults-guidance-for-prescribing-exercise.

Ashworth, N. L., Chad, K. E., Harrison, E. L., Reeder, B. A., and Marshall, S. C. (2005). Home versus center based physical activity programs in older adults. *Cochrane Database of Systematic Reviews,* Issue 1. Art. No.: CD004017. DOI: 10.1002/14651858. CD004017.pub2.

Bandura, A. (1997). *Self-efficacy: The exercise of control.* New York: W.H. Freeman.

Bandura, A. (2001). Social cognitive theory: An agentic perspective. *Annual Review of Psychology, 52,* 1-26.

Baranowski, T., Anderson, C., and Carmack, C. (1998). Mediating variable framework in physical activity interventions. How are we doing? How might we do better? *American Journal of Preventive Medicine, 15*, 260-297.

Berger, B. G., Pargman, D., and Weinberg, R. S. (2002). *Foundations of exercise psychology.* Morgantown, WV: Fitness Information Technology.

Biddle, S. J. H. (1999). Motivation and perceptions of control: Tracing its development and plotting its future in exercise and sport psychology. *Journal of Sport and Exercise Psychology, 21*, 1-23.

Blanchard, C. M., Fortier, M., Sweet, S., O'Sullivan, T., Hogg, W., Reid, R. D., et al. (2007). Explaining physical activity levels from a self-efficacy perspective: The physical activity counseling trial. *Annals of Behavioral Medicine, 34*, 323-328.

Buckworth, J., and Dishman, R. K. (2002). *Exercise psychology*. Champaign, IL: Human Kinetics.

Bunke, S., Apitzsch, E., and Baeckstroem, M. (2013). The impact of social influence on physical activity among adolescents: A longitudinal study. *European Journal of Sport Science, 13,* 86-95.

Burke, S. M., Carron, A. V., Eys, M. A., Ntoumanis, N., and Estabrooks, P. A. (2006). Group versus individual approach: A meta-analysis of the effectiveness of interventions to promote physical activity. *Sport and Exercise Psychology Review, 2,* 19-35.

Cameron, C., Wolfe, R., and Craig, C. L. (2007). *Physical activity and sport: Encouraging children to be active.* Ottawa, ON: Canadian Fitness and Lifestyle Research Institute: Retrieved September 23, 2011 from http://www.cflri.ca.

Canadian Society for Exercise Physiology. (2011). *Canadian physical activity guidelines.* Retrieved September 6, 2011 from http://www.csep.ca/english/view.asp?x=804.

Cao, D. S., Lippke, S., and Wei, L. (2011). The importance of autonomous regulation for students' successful translation of intentions into behavior changes via planning. *Advances in Preventive Medicine.* Article ID 697856, 6 pages.

Cao, D. S., Schuez, N., Xie, G. R., and Lippke, S. (2013). Planning skills moderate the intention-planning cognitions-behaviour relation: A longitudinal study on physical activity in Chinese adolescents. *Research in Sports Medicine, 21,* 12-23.

Carron, A. V., Hausenblas, H. A., and Mack, D. (1996). Social influence and exercise: A meta-analysis. *Journal of Sport and Exercise Psychology, 18*, 1-16.

Centers for Disease Control and Prevention. (2000). *National health and nutrition examination survey.* Atlanta, GA: US Department of Health and Human Services, Centers for Disease Control and Prevention, National Center for Health Statistics.

Center for Disease Control and Prevention. *Exercise.* Retrieved September 6, 2011 from http://www.cdc.gov/physicalactivity/everyone/glossary.

Chatzisarantis, N. L. D, and Hagger, M. S. (2005). Effects of a brief intervention based on the theory of planned behavior on leisure-time physical activity participation. *Journal of Sport and Exercise Psychology, 27,* 470-487.

Courneya, K. S. (1995). Understanding readiness for regular physical activity in older individuals: An application of the theory of planned behavior. *Health Psychology, 14*, 80-87.

Cox, M. H. (1984). Fitness and lifestyle-programs for business and industry: Problems in recruitment and retention. *Journal of Cardiac Rehabilitation, 4*, 136-142.

Cress, M. E., Buchner, D. M., Prochaska, T., Rimmer, J., Brown, M., Macera, C., et al., (2005). Best practices for physical activity programs and behavior counseling in older adult populations. *Journal of Aging and Physical Activity, 13*, 61-74.

Dawson, K. A., and Brawley, L. R. (2000). Examining the relationship between exercise goals, self-efficacy, and overt behaviors with beginning exercisers. *Journal of Applied Social Psychology, 30*, 315-329.

Dawson, K. A., Brawley, L. R., and Maddux, J. E. (2000). Examining the relationships among concepts of control and exercise attendance. *Journal of Sport and Exercise Psychology, 22*, 131-144.

Dawson, K. A., Robertson-Wilson, J., and Martin Ginis, K. (2011). Physical activity interventions. In P. Crocker (2nd Ed.). *Sport and exercise psychology: A Canadian perspective,* (pp. 337-362). Toronto, ON: Pearson Canada.

Dawson, K. A., Tracey, J., and Berry, T. (2008). Evaluation of work place group and internet based physical activity interventions on psychological variables associated with exercise behavior. *Journal of Sports Science and Medicine, 7*, 537-543.

de Bruijn, G-J., Verkooijen, K., de Vries, N. K., and van den Putte, B. (2012). Antecedents of self identity and consequences for action control: An application of the theory of planned behaviour in the exercise domain. *Psychology of Sport and Exercise, 13,* 771-778.

Desharnais, R., Bouillon, J., and Godin, G. (1986). Self-efficacy and outcome expectations as determinants of exercise adherence. *Psychological Reports, 59*, 1155-1159.

Dishman, R. K. (Ed.) (1994). *Advances in exercise adherence*. Champaign, IL: Human Kinetics.

Dishman, R. K., and Duckworth, J. (1998). Exercise psychology. In J. P. Williams (Ed.), *Applied sport psychology: Personal growth to peak performance,* (pp. 445-464). London, UK: Mayfield.

Dishman, R. K., and Sallis, J. F. (1994). Determinants and interventions for physical activity and exercise. In C. Bouchard, R. J. Shephard, and T. Stephens (Eds.), *Physical activity, fitness, and health: International proceedings and consensus statement* (pp. 214-238). Champaign IL: Human Kinetics Press.

DuCharme, K. A., and Brawley, L. R. (1995). Predicting the intentions and behavior of exercise initiates using two forms of self-efficacy. *Journal of Behavioral Medicine, 18*, 479-497.

DuCharme, K. A., Widmeyer, W. N., Dorsch, K., and Hoar, S. (1996). The relationship of social support and self-efficacy to exercise intentions and attendance at a private fitness club. *Journal of Sport and Exercise Psychology, 18*, 27-36.

Duncan, T. E., and McAuley, E. (1993). Social support and efficacy cognitions in exercise adherence: A latent growth analysis. *Journal of Behavioral Medicine, 16,* 199-217.

Duncan, T. E., McAuley, E., Stoolmiller, M., and Duncan, S. C. (1993). Serial fluctuations in exercise behavior as a function of social support and efficacy cognitions. *Journal of Applied Social Psychology, 23*, 1498-1522.

Evers, A., Klusmann, V., Schwarzer, R., and Heuser, I. (2011). Adherence to physical and mental activity interventions: Coping plans as a mediator and prior adherence as a moderator. *British Journal of Health Psychology, 17,* 477-491.

Evers, A., Klusmann, V., Ziegelmann, J. P., Schwarzer, R., and Heuser, I. (2012). Long-term adherence to a physical activity intervention: The role of telephone-assisted vs. self-administered coping plans and strategy use. *Psychology and Health, 27,* 784-797.

Exercise Is Medicine. Retrieved February 7, 2012 from www.exerciseismedicine.org.

Fishbein, M., and Ajzen, I. (1975). *Belief, attitude, intention, and behavior: An introduction to theory and research.* Reading, MA: Addison-Wesley.

Fleig, L., Lippke, S., Pomp, S., and Schwarzer, R. (2011). Intervention effects of exercise self-regulation on physical activity and eating fruits and vegetables: A longitudinal study in orthopedic and cardiac rehabilitation. *Preventive Medicine, 53,* 182-187.

Fraser, S. H., and Rodgers, W. M. (2012). The influence of general and exercise specific social support on self-efficacy for overcoming barriers to cardiac rehabilitation. *Journal of Applied Social Psychology, 42,* 1811-1829.

Frederickson, B. F. (2001). The role of positive emotions in positive psychology: The broaden-and-build theory of positive emotions. *American Psychologist, 56,* 218-226.

Fuchs, R., Seelig, H., Goehner, W., Burton, N. W., and Brown, W. J. (2012). Cognitive mediation of intervention effects on physical exercise: Causal models for the adoption and maintenance stage. *Psychology and Health, 27,* 1480-1499.

Garcia, A. W., and King, A. C. (1991). Predicting long-term adherence to aerobic exercise: A comparison of two models. *Journal of Sport and Exercise Psychology, 13*, 394-410.

Gellert, P., Ziegelmann, J. P., Lippke, S., and Schwarzer, R. (2012). Future time perspective and health behaviors: Temporal framing of self-regulatory processes in physical exercise and dietary behaviors. *Annals of Behavioral Medicine, 43,* 203-218.

Gellert, P., Ziegelmann, J. P., and Schwarzer, R. (2012). Affective and health-related outcome expectancies for physical activity in older adults. *Psychology and Health, 27,* 816-828.

Gollwitzer, P. M. (1999). Implementation intentions: Strong effects of simple plans. *American Psychologist, 54*, 493-503.

Gruber, K. J. (2008). Social support for exercise and dietary habits among college students. *Adolescence, 43,* 557-576.

Hall, P. A., Fong, G. T., and Cheng, A. Y. (2012). Time perspective and weight management behaviors in newly diagnosed Type 2 diabetes: A meditational analysis. *Journal of Behavioral Medicine, 35,* 569-580.

Hankonen, N., Pilvikki, A., Ghisletta, P., Renner, B., and Uutela, A. (2010). Gender differences in social cognitive determinants of exercise adoption. *Psychology and Health, 25,* 55-69.

Haskell, W. L., Lee, I., Pate, R. R., Powell, K. E., Blair, S. N., Franklin, B. A., et al. (2007). Physical activity and public health: Updated recommendation for adults from the American College of Sports Medicine and the American Health Association. *Medicine and Science in Sports and Exercise, 39, 1423-1434.*

Hobbs, N., Dixon, D., Johnston, M., and Howie, K. (2013). Can the theory of planned behaviour predict the physical activity behavior of individuals? *Psychology and Health, 28,* 234-249.

Hsiao, E. T., and Thayer, R. E. (1997). Exercising for mood regulation: The importance of experience. *Personality and Individual Differences, 24*, 829-836.

Hu, L., Motl, R. W., McAuley, E., and Konopack, J. F. (2007). Effects of self-efficacy on physical activity enjoyment of college-aged women. *International Journal of Behavioral Medicine, 14,* 92-96.

Jackson, B., Whipp, P. R., Chua, K. L. P., Dimmock, J. A., and Hagger, M. S. (2013). Students' tripartite efficacy beliefs in high school physical education: Within-and cross-domain relations with motivational processes and leisure-time physical activity. *Journal of Sport and Exercise Psychology, 35,* 72-84.

Kasimatis, M., Miller, M., and Marcussen, L. (1996). The effects of implicit theories on exercise motivation. *Journal of Research in Personality, 30,* 510-516.

Kavussanu, M., and McAuley, E. (1995). Exercise and optimism: Are highly active individuals more optimistic? *Journal of Sport and Exercise Psychology, 17,* 246-258.

King, A. C., Haskell, W. L., Young, D. R., Oka, R. K., and Stefanick, M. L. (1995). Long-term effects of varying intensities and formats of physical activity on participation rates, fitness, and lipoproteins in men and women aged 50 to 65 years. *Circulation, 9,* 2596-2604.

King, A. C., Kiernan, M., Oman, R. F., Kraemer, H. C., Hull, M., and Ahn, D. (1997). Can we identify who will adhere to long-term physical activity? Signal detection methodology as a potential aid to clinical decision making. *Health Psychology, 16,* 380-389.

King, A. C., Taylor, C. B., Haskell, W. L., and DeBusk, R. F. (1990). Identifying strategies for increasing employee physical activity levels: Findings from the Stanford/Lockheed exercise survey. *Health Psychology, 17,* 269-285.

Koring, M., Richert, J., Parschau, L., Ernsting, A., Lippke, S., and Schwarzer, R. (2012). A combined planning and self-efficacy intervention to promote physical activity: Effectiveness and working mechanisms? *Psychology, Health and Medicine, 17,* 488-498.

Lee, C. (1993). Attitudes, knowledge, and stages of change: A survey of exercise patterns in older Australian women. *Health Psychology, 12,* 476-480.

Lewis, M. A., and Rook, K. S. (1999). Social control in personal relationships: Impact on health behaviors and psychological distress. *Health Psychology, 18,* 63-71.

Lippke, S., and Plotnikoff, R. C. (2013). Testing two principles of the health action process approach in individuals with type 2 diabetes. *Health Psychology.* doi: 10.1037/a0030182

Lippke, S., Schwarzer, R., Ziegelmann, J. P., Scholz, U., and Schulz, B. (2010). Testing stage-specific effects of a stage-matched intervention: A randomized controlled trial targeting physical exercise and its predictors. *Health Education and Behavior, 37,* 533-546.

Lochbaum, M. R., Rhodes, R. E., Stevenson, S. J., Surles, J., Stevens, T., and Wang, C. K. J. (2010). Does gender moderate the exercising personality? An examination of continuous and stage-based exercise. *Psychology, health and medicine, 15,* 50-60.

Locke, E. A., and Latham, G. P. (2002). Building a practical useful theory of goal setting and task motivation. *American Psychologist, 57,* 705-717.

Lombard, D. N., Lombard, T. N., and Winett, R. A. (1995). Walking to meet health guidelines: The effect of prompting frequency and prompt structure. *Health Psychology, 14,* 164-170.

Lox, C., Martin Ginis, K. A., and Petruzzello, S. J. (2010). *The psychology of exercise: Integrating theory and practice.* Scottsdale, AZ: Holcomb Hathaway Publishers.

Luszczynska, A., Mazurkiewicz, M., Ziegelmann, J. P., and Schwarzer, R. (2007). Recovery self-efficacy and intention as predictors of running or jogging behavior: A cross-lagged panel analysis over a two-year period. *Psychology of Sport and Exercise, 8,* 247-260.

Luszczynska, A., Schwarzer, R., Lippke, S., and Mazurkiewicz, M. (2011). Self-efficacy as a moderator of the planning-behavior relationship in interventions designed to promote physical activity. *Psychology and Health, 26,* 151-166.

Maddux, J. E. (1993). Social cognitive models of health and exercise behavior: An introduction and review of conceptual issues. *Journal of Applied Sport Psychology, 5,* 116-140.

Maddux, J. E. (1999). Expectancies and the social-cognitive perspective: Basic principles, processes, and variables. In I. Kirsch (Ed.), *How expectancies shape experience* (pp. 17-40). Washington, DC: American Psychological Association.

Maddux, J. E. (2007). Expectancies and health behavior: Basic principles, processes, and variables. In S. Ayers, A. Baum, C. McManus, S. Newman, K. Wallston, J. Weinman, and R. West (Eds.), *Cambridge handbook of psychology, health, and medicine* (2nd ed., pp. 87-91). Cambridge, UK: Cambridge University Press.

Maddux, J. E. (2009). Self-regulation. In S. J. Lopez (Ed.), *Encyclopedia of positive psychology* (p. 874). New York, NY: Blackwell Publishing.

Maddux, J. E. (2010). Social cognitive theories and clinical interventions: Basic principles and guidelines. In J. E. Maddux and J. P. Tangney (Eds.), *Social psychological foundations of clinical psychology* (pp. 395-415). New York: Guilford.

Maddux, J. E., and Rogers, R. W. (1983). Protection motivation and self-efficacy: A revised theory of fear appeals and attitude change. *Journal of Experimental Social Psychology, 19,* 469-479.

Malina, R. M. (1996). Tracking of physical activity and physical fitness across the lifespan. *Research Quarterly for Exercise and Sport, 57,* 48-57.

Marcus, B. H., Dubbert, P. M., Forsyth, L. H., McKenzie, T. L., Stone, E. J., Dunn, A. L., et al. (2000). Physical activity behavior change: Issues in adoption and maintenance. *Health Psychology, 19,* 32-41.

McAuley, E., and Courneya, K. S. (1993). Adherence to exercise and physical activity as health-promoting behaviors: Attitudinal and self-efficacy influences. *Applied and Preventive Psychology, 2,* 65-77.

Nied, R. J., and Franklin, B. (2002). Promoting and prescribing exercise for the elderly. *American Family Physician, 65,* 419-427.

Oettingen, G., and Gollwitzer, P. M. (2010). Strategies of setting and implementing goals: Mental contrasting and implementation intentions. In J. E. Maddux and J. P. Tangney (Eds.), *Social psychological foundations of clinical psychology* (pp. 114-135). New York: Guilford.

Oka, R. K., King, A. C., and Young, D. R. (1995). Sources of social support as predictors of exercise adherence in women and men ages 50 to 65 years. *Women's Health: Research on Gender, Behavior, and Policy, 1,* 161-175.

Oman, R. F., and King, A. C. (2000). The effect of life events and exercise program format on the adoption and maintenance of exercise behavior. *Health Psychology, 19,* 605-612.

Orbell, S., and Verplanken, B. (2010). The automatic component of habit in health behavior: Habit as cue-contingent automaticity. *Health Psychology, 29,* 374-383.

Peterson, L. R., Clark, M. M., Novotny, P., Kung, S., Sloan, J. A., Patten, C. A., et al. (2008). Relationship of optimism-pessimism and health-related quality of life in breast cancer survivors. *Journal of Psychosocial Oncology, 26,* 15-32.

Plotnikoff, R. C., Lubans, D. R., Trinh, L., and Craig, C. L. (2012). A 15-year longitudinal test of the theory of planned behavior to predict physical activity in a randomized sample of Canadian adults. *Psychology of Sport and Exercise, 13,* 521-527.

Pomp, S., Fleig, L., Schwarzer, R., and Lippke, S. (2012). Effects of a self-regulation intervention on exercise are moderated by depressive symptoms: A quasi-experimental study. *International Journal of Clinical and Health Psychology, 13,* 1-8.

Prestwick, A., Lawton, R., and Conner, M. (2003). The use of implementation intentions and the decision balance sheet in promoting exercise behavior. *Psychology and Health, 18,* 707-721.

Prochaska, J. O., and Prochaska, J. M. (2010). Self-directed change: A transtheoretical model. In J. E. Maddux and J. P. Tangney (Eds.), *Social psychological foundations of clinical psychology* (pp. 431-440). New York: Guilford.

Reed, J. A., and Phillips, D. A. (2005). Relationships between physical activity and the proximity of exercise facilities and home exercise equipment used by undergraduate university students. *Journal of American College Health, 53,* 285-290.

Rhodes, R. E., Fiala, B., and Nasuti, G. (2012). Action control of exercise behavior: Evaluation of social cognition, cross-behavioral regulation, and automaticity. *Behavioral Medicine, 38,* 121-128.

Rogers, R. W. (1975). A protection motivation theory of fear appeals and attitude change. *Journal of Psychology, 91,* 93-114.

Rogers, R. W., and Prentice-Dunn, S. (1997). Protection motivation theory. In D. Gochman (Ed.), *Handbook of health behavior research: Personal and social determinants,* (Vol 1, pp. 113-132). New York: Plenum.

Rothman, A. J. (2000). Toward a theory-based analysis of behavioral maintenance. *Health Psychology, 19,* 64-69.

Saklofske, D. H., Austin, E. J., and Rohr, B. A. (2006). Personality, emotional intelligence and exercise. *Journal of Health Psychology, 12,* 937-948.

Sallis, J. F., and Owen, N. (1999). *Physical activity and behavioral medicine.* Newbury Park, CA: Sage.

Sallis, J. F., Prochaska, J. J., Taylor, W. C., Hill, J. O., and Geraci, J. C. (1999). Correlates of physical activity in a national sample of girls and boys in grades 4 through 12. *Health Psychology, 18,* 410-415.

Schwarzer, R. (2008). Modeling health behavior change: How to predict and modify the adoption and maintenance of health behaviors. *Applied Psychology: An International Review, 57,* 1-29.

Stephens, T., and Craig, A. V. (1990). *The well-being of Canadians: Highlights of the 1988 Campbell's Survey.* Ottawa, Canada: Canadian Fitness and Lifestyle Research Institute.

Stephens, T., Jacobs, D. R., and White, C. C. (1985). A descriptive epidemiology of leisure-time activity. *Public Health Reports, 100,* 147-158.

Stetson, B. A., Rahn, J. M., Dubbert, P. M., Wilner, B. I., and Mercury, M. G. (1997). Prospective evaluation of the effects of stress on exercise adherence in community-residing women. *Health Psychology, 16,* 515-520.

Strecher, V. J., Champion, V. L., and Rosenstock, I. M. (1997). The health belief model and health behavior. In D. Gochman (Ed.), *Handbook of health behavior research: Personal and social determinants* (Vol 1, pp. 71-92). New York: Plenum.

Tkachuk, G. A., and Martin, G. L. (1999). Exercise therapy for patients with psychiatric disorders: Research and clinical applications. *Professional Psychology: Research and Practice, 30*, 275-282.

Tracey, J., Dawson, K., and Berry, T. (2009). Participant experiences in a group or internet-based physical activity intervention. *Malaysian Journal of Sport Science and Recreation, 4*, 11-30.

Tucker, J. S., and Mueller, J. S. (2000). Spouses' social control of health behaviors: Use and effectiveness of specific strategies. *Personality and Social Psychology Bulletin, 26,* 1120-1130.

United States Department of Health and Human Services (1996). *Physical activity and health: A report of the Surgeon General.* Atlanta, GA: US Department of Health and Human Services, Centers for Disease Control and Prevention: National Center for Chronic Disease Prevention and Health Promotion.

Vallance, J. K., Lavallee, C., Culos-Reed, N. S., and Trudeau, M. G. (2012). Predictors of physical activity among rural and small town breast cancer survivors: An application of the theory of planned beaviour. *Psychology, Health, and Medicine, 17,* 685-697.

Wankel, L. M. (1985). Personal and situational factors affecting exercise involvement: The importance of enjoyment. *Research Quarterly for Exercise and Sport, 56*, 275-282.

Wankel, L. M. (1987). Enhancing motivation for involvement in voluntary exercise programs. In M. L. Maher (Ed.). *Advances in motivation and achievement: Enhancing motivation* (pp. 239-286). Greenwich, CT: JAI Press.

Warburton, D. E. R., Nicol, C. W., and Bredin, S. S. D. (2006). Health benefits of physical activity: The evidence. *Canadian Medical Association Journal, 174,* 801-809.

Wiedemann, A. U., Lippke, S., Reuter, T., Ziegelmann, J. P., and Schulz, B. (2010). The more the better? The number of plans predicts health behavior. *Applied Psychology: Health and Well-Being, 3,* 87-106.

Wiedemann, A. U., Lippke, S., and Schwarzer, R. (2011). Multiple plans and memory performance: Results of a randomized control trial targeting fruit and vegetable intake. *Journal of Behavioral Medicine, 35*(4), 387-392.

Willis, J. D., and Campbell, L. F. (1992). *Exercise psychology.* Champaign, IL: Human Kinetics.

Witte, K., and Allen, M. (2000). A meta-analysis of fear appeals: Implications for effective public health campaigns. *Health Education and Behavior, 27,* 591-615.

World Health Organization. http://www.who.int/topics/physical_activity/en/ (retrieved July 24, 2013).

In: Positive Human Functioning ... Volume 2 ISBN: 978-1-62948-973-5
Editors: A. R. Gomes, R. Resende and A. Albuquerque © 2014 Nova Science Publishers, Inc.

Chapter 7

SOCIAL FACTORS IN EXERCISE SETTINGS

Kimberley L. Gammage and Larkin Lamarche
Department of Kinesiology, Brock University, St. Catharines, Ontario, Canada

ABSTRACT

In this chapter, we provide evidence of the important influence social factors have on positive human development within a physical activity context. Specifically, we discuss *empirical and conceptual findings* for three main areas of research. First, we examine the literature regarding social support – the types and sources of social support, outcomes related to social support, how social support positively impacts such outcomes, and social support in special populations. Second, we summarize literature with respect to a specific type of social influence: cohesion. In this section we present evidence of the link between cohesion and adherence as well as other outcomes, and provide insight into teambuilding as a method to enhance cohesion and subsequent outcomes. The last topic we discuss is group-related factors in exercise. We summarize research on two types of exercise leaders (group fitness instructors and personal trainers), and discuss important qualities of the exercise leader that have been shown to be influential (leadership style, experience, and physical characteristics). In addition, we examine literature on characteristics of the exercise group (i.e., co-exercisers' characteristics, group atmosphere, and group size). We have also included a section on *practical implications* regarding social factors in a physical activity context. We conclude the chapter with *key points* that highlight future directions in the research area of social factors in exercise settings.

INTRODUCTION

Despite the numerous physical and psychological benefits of regular physical activity, the majority of individuals remain inactive or insufficiently active to experience the positive benefits of regular physical activity. This chapter will present evidence that social factors are important influences to consider when promoting exercise participation. We first discuss social support as a primary form of social influence. We then discuss cohesion as an important type of social influence in exercise. Our third topic is group-related factors, such as exercise leaders and group characteristics. We end the chapter with practical implications and key points.

Social Influences in Exercise

Alcock, Carment, and Sadava (1991) defined social influence as perceptions of pressure (real or imagined) from others to change behavior, attitudes or beliefs. Social influences are positively related to physical and mental health (Thoits, 2011 for review), and exercise is one setting in which they may be particularly important.

Franklin (1988) outlined several factors that influence adherence to exercise programs. Many were forms of social influence (e.g., group camaraderie, leadership, spouse support, peer approval). He specifically noted that exercising alone was a predictor of drop-out. Since then, the importance of social factors in exercise settings has consistently been shown. In their meta-analysis, Carron, Hausenblas, and Mack (1996) concluded that, depending on the specific nature of the social influence, small to large effects were found on adherence as well as cognitive and affective outcomes of exercise. Numerous reviews (e.g., Sallis, Prochaska, and Taylor, 2000; Trost, Owen, Bauman, Sallis, and Brown, 2002) have reported social influences as important correlates of physical activity behavior across a variety of populations.

Preferences for Exercise Context

Research has examined exercise context preferences (Burke, Carron, and Eys, 2006; King, Haskell, Taylor, Kraemer, and DeBusk, 1991; King et al., 2000; Wilcox, King, Brassington, and Ahn, 1999). Some individuals prefer to exercise alone versus in a group (King et al., 1991; Wilcox et al., 1999) and have rated exercising alone as more appealing than exercising in a group (King et al., 2000). However, these studies investigated preferences for exercising alone or with others only (Burke, Carron, and Shapcott, 2008). Burke, Carron, and Eys (2006) examined a greater variety of settings and found that undergraduate students most preferred to do aerobic exercise with others but outside of a structured class. In fact, women rated exercising completely alone as the least preferred exercise context. Beauchamp, Carron, McCutcheon, and Harper (2007) also concluded that the majority of people prefer to exercise with others compared to completely alone.

Effectiveness of Exercising in Difference Contexts

In a meta-analysis, Burke, Carron, Eys, Ntoumanis, and Estabrooks (2006) compared the effectiveness of exercising in a home-based program with no contact from researchers or health-care professionals, a home-based program that involved some contact, standard exercise classes, and exercise classes where principles of group dynamics were implemented to increase group cohesion. They found that exercising in a true group was superior to a standard exercise class, which did not differ from exercise in a home-based program with contact. Exercising at home without contact was least effective. Given individual preferences and greater effectiveness arising from exercising with others, examining social influences is important and may provide ways to increase adherence.

CONCEPTUAL AND EMPIRICAL FINDINGS REGARDING SOCIAL SUPPORT IN EXERCISE

Social Networks

One approach to examining the influence of others has been to examine the impact of social networks on exercise. Social networks are structural units that describe an individual's social ties and relationships, including factors such as the number or closeness of social ties, the interconnectedness between ties, or an individual's location within the social network (Gottlieb and Bergen, 2010). Generally, there is similarity in physical activity levels within peer and friendship groups, particularly for high intensity physical activity (Macdonald-Wallis, Jago, Page, Brockman, and Thompson, 2011; Macdonald-Wallis, Jago, and Sterne, 2012). Voorhees et al. (2005) also found that the nature of the social relationships was important; the frequency of a best friend's physical activity was a better predictor of physical activity level than the number of active friends.

Social Support Defined

Social support is a specific type of social influence defined as any perceived or real assistance provided by others, with the intent to help people perform a behavior or achieve a goal (Duncan, Duncan, and Strycker, 2005; Gottlieb and Bergen, 2010; Thoits, 2011). Thus, social support for physical activity is any attempt by others to help people be physically active.

Types of Social Support

Although many types of social support have been identified, there are 3 main categories: emotional, informational, and instrumental (Helgeson and Cohen, 1996). These types of social support are relevant in physical activity settings (Taylor, Baranowski, and Sallis, 1994). *Emotional support* refers to verbal and non-verbal encouragement and caring. Congratulating a spouse for going to the gym, sympathizing with a friend after a challenging workout, listening to a friend talk about her accomplishments training for a marathon, or encouraging a child to try a new activity are all examples of emotional support. *Informational support* includes advice, instructions, or directions about how to be active. For instance, a doctor providing a patient with information about how much exercise to perform, a personal trainer giving instructions on correct technique, or a friend providing advice on how to fit exercise into a busy lifestyle are all informational support. Finally, *instrumental support* refers to tangible assistance for physical activity participation. Parents driving their kids to games, children cooking dinner one night a week so their mother can go to the gym after work, or a wife buying her husband a bike for his birthday so he can cycle to work are all examples of instrumental support.

Sources of Social Support

The source of social support – or who is providing that support – is also an important consideration. Family, friends and peers, and experts (healthcare providers, fitness leaders, or physical education teachers) can all provide any type of social support. These sources of social support can be important at various times throughout the life. For children, family – especially parents – is most important (Robbins, Stommel, and Hamel, 2008). In adolescents, peers become relatively more influential (Prochaska, Rodgers and Sallis, 2002). Through adulthood and older adulthood, sources such as spouses and doctors increase in importance (Schutzer and Graves, 2004). Whatever the source and type, it is clear that social support is an important consideration when understanding physical activity behavior.

Outcomes of Social Support in Exercise

Research has focused on whether social support can help to increase physical activity participation and adherence in a variety of samples. Consistently, greater perceptions of social support (across type and source) are associated with better adherence to physical activity (see Bauman et al., 2012; Sallis et al., 2000; Trost et al., 2002 for reviews). For example, Trost et al. (2002) found social support from family, friends, and staff/instructors was strongly positively related to exercise behavior, while lack of social support was negatively related to physical activity in adults. In children and adolescents, Sallis et al. (2000) found that parental social support, support from significant others, and direct assistance from parents were all positively associated with physical activity in adolescents. In children, findings were more varied, but encouragement was positively associated with physical activity. Most recently, Bauman and colleagues (2012) examined systematic reviews of correlates of physical activity and concluded that social support was a correlate of physical activity across the lifespan.

One of the limitations noted in this research is that studies often do not distinguish between types or sources of social support that may be important; these factors change across the lifespan. For example, in older adults, non-family members are important sources of social support (Clark, Patrick, and Grembowski, 1995; Eyler et al., 1999; Wolinsky, Stump, and Clark, 1995). Wolinsky et al. (1995) found that non-family social support (but not family social support) was positively related to regular physical activity. For older adults, healthcare providers (e.g., doctors) are important and preferred sources of social support (Balde, Figueras, Hawkins, and Miller, 2003; Schutzer and Graves, 2004; Wilson and Spink, 2006). By contrast, Resnick, Orwig, Magaziner, and Wynne (2002) found that social support from friends (but not family or experts such as physicians) was associated indirectly with physical activity behavior.

During childhood and adolescence, a very different picture of social support emerges. Generally, during childhood, parents are the most important sources of social support for physical activity (Beets, Cardinal, and Alderman, 2010; Robbins et al., 2008; Sallis et al., 2000). In their review of parental social support for physical activity in youth, Beets et al. (2010) found that tangible support (such as transportation, paying for fees, or buying equipment) was positively related to children's physical activity levels. Further, being physically active with children, watching children be active, and encouragement were all associated with increased intensity and frequency of physical activity (Beets et al., 2010).

In middle school children (age 10-14 years), parents, friends/peers, and coaches/teachers were all important sources of social support, with father support the best predictor of physical activity (Duncan et al., 2005; Robbins et al., 2008). Further, being physically active with children, watching children be active (without participating themselves), and encouragement have all been associated with increased intensity and frequency of physical activity (Duncan et al., 2005; Robbins et al., 2008).

In adolescents, perceived encouragement from parents and friends was positively related to after-school physical activity, while encouragement from friends was associated with lunchtime physical activity and active transportation (Hohepa, Scragg, Schofield, Kolt, and Schaaf, 2007). These findings are consistent with Prochaska et al. (2002) who reported peer support to be most strongly related to physical activity in adolescents. These findings suggest that the relative importance of the types and sources of social support change across the lifespan.

How Does Social Support Work?

One of the most consistent findings in the literature is that social support does not directly affect levels of physical activity. Rather, self-efficacy mediates the relationship between social support and physical activity – that is, social support increases self-efficacy, which in turns leads to greater physical activity (Duncan and McAuley, 1993). This finding has been replicated in adolescents (Beets, Pitetti, and Forlaw, 2007; Motl, Dishman, Saunders, Dowda, and Pate, 2007), university students (Rovniak, Anderson, Winett, and Stephens, 2002), middle-aged adults (Ayotte, Margrett, and Hicks-Patrick, 2010; Duncan and McAuley, 1993) and older adults (Ayotte et al., 2010; Resnick et al., 2002). A second potential mediator of the social support-physical activity relationship is self-regulation (Anderson, Worcik, Winett, and Williams, 2006; Ayotte et al., 2010), which refers to behaviors, such as goal-setting or planning, that enable people to control and manage their motivation and behaviors (Bandura, 1997, 2005). Social support led to increased perceptions of self-regulation, which in turn was associated with higher levels of physical activity in adults and older adults.

Other Outcomes of Social Support in Physical Activity Settings

Social support has also been linked to many other positive outcomes such as subjective well-being, and perceptions of the overall goodness of one's life (Lehnert, Sudeck, and Conselmann, 2012; McAuley et al., 2000). For example, in older adults, McAuley, Elavsky, Jerome, Konopack, and Marquez (2005) found that higher initial social support during two types of exercise interventions (walking and stretching/toning) was associated with higher positive well-being at the end of the first month of exercise. In the same participants, McAuley et al. (2000) found that increases in social support were associated with increases in life satisfaction over the 6 months of an exercise intervention and during a 6-month follow-up.

Qualitative research with older adults has also provided evidence of the benefits of social support on other psychological outcomes. For example, in participants enrolled in group-based exercise program (compared to a home-based program), perceptions of social support were associated with enjoyment and reduced perceptions of barriers to exercise. Participants also indicated that they enjoyed the opportunity for interaction, as it provided motivation to exercise compared to the home-based program (Fox, Stathi, McKenna, and Davis, 2007).

In adults, social support has also been related to positive psychological outcomes. In a qualitative study with adults aged 19-32 years, social support was associated with increased levels of comfort, fewer negative emotions, less self-consciousness, higher enjoyment, and greater focus on their workout (Pridgeon and Grogan, 2012). It was also reported to be helpful for maintaining motivation to go to the gym through increases in self-efficacy. Men reported that emotional support from other men led to feelings of belonging and acceptance, and increased self-esteem and self-identity. Women reported that an exercise partner made them feel less intimidated, less self-conscious, and more empowered and confident while at the gym.

In adolescents, exercise-related social support has been associated with positive affect. Two types of social support provided by peers (esteem support, in which friends believe they are competent at physical activity, and companionship) were associated with positive affect in physical activity (Duncan, 1993). Beets et al. (2010) reported that in girls, social support from parents was associated with increased attraction to physical activity and higher perceived competence.

Social Support for Physical Activity in Special Populations

The majority of social support research has examined healthy populations. However, there is also evidence that special populations benefit from social support.

Cardiac Rehabilitation

Much of the earliest work on social support for physical activity comes from the literature on cardiac rehabilitation. Social support has been positively related to adherence in cardiac rehabilitation settings (Dracup, 1994; Erling and Oldridge, 1985), with spousal support particularly effective. For example, Erling and Oldridge (1985) found that 33% of their participants who attended without their spouse dropped out compared to a 10% dropout rate for participants who attended with their spouse. Further, 65% of spouses perceived that patients' psychological health improved and 48% perceived their social adjustment improved. Interestingly, the spouses also reported a decrease in their anxiety about the patient's exercise program. Type of support is also important in this setting. Fraser and Rodgers (2012) found that exercise specific support, designed to help people be active, and general emotional support were associated with lower stress and higher self-efficacy for exercise.

Breast Cancer

The importance of social support for physical activity has been investigated in breast cancer survivors. Dragon boat racing has become a popular activity for women recovering from breast cancer, providing them with a safe, effective form of physical activity following treatment. Research examining women's perceptions of dragon boating has found that social support is consistently reported by women (Unruh and Elvin, 2004). Many women report that they join dragon boating for fun and fitness, without social support being the focus of attention (McDonough, Sabiston, and Crocker, 2008; McDonough, Sabiston, and Ullrich-French, 2011). While social support benefits were not expected they did occur over the season (McDonough et al., 2011), with women stating that they did not realize until after they received social support that they were missing it and that it was important (McDonough et al., 2008).

Emotional and informational social support (including empowerment, encouragement, information and other resources, and humor) are important in this context and develop over time (McDonough et al., 2008; Parry, 2007, 2008). All types of social support were linked to psychosocial well-being, a sense of belonging, and reductions in stress in survivors (Sabiston, McDonough, and Crocker, 2007). Women also noted that being able to provide social support to others was important (McDonough et al., 2011; Sabiston et al., 2007).

Neurological Disorders

Social support for physical activity for individuals with neurological disorders such as Parkinson's disease and multiple sclerosis has also been demonstrated. Ravenek and Schneider (2009) found that patients reported receiving instrumental (e.g., transportation), informational (e.g., advice from a neurologist to be active) and emotional (e.g., phone calls from friends) support from family, friends, co-workers, health-care professionals, and support groups. Social support was associated with increases in self-efficacy and intention to exercise, which in turn led to higher beliefs that the disease could be managed through physical activity. Motl, Snook, McAuley, Scott, and Douglass (2006) examined correlates of physical activity in patients with multiple sclerosis, and found that social support was significantly related to self-efficacy, which in turn predicted physical activity behavior. Social support has also been linked with quality of life. Physical activity led to increased feelings of social support, which in turn was associated with higher quality of life (Motl, McAuley, and Snook, 2007; Motl, McAuley, Snook, and Gliottoni, 2009). Motl and McAuley (2009) also found that changes in physical activity were indirectly associated with changes in quality of life, through several variables including social support.

Physical Disabilities

In their study examining motivators and barriers to physical activity in those with a physical disability, Junker and Carlberg (2011) reported that social support specifically from family and friends was significant. Along with an accessible environment, having an instructor who could adapt exercises to be appropriate was the most important factor in helping them to be physically active. Rimmer, Riley, Wang, Rauworth, and Jurkowski (2004) similarly found that a lack of knowledge from fitness professionals on how to adapt exercises, lack of information on facilities that were accessible, and lack of support from family and friends were the biggest barriers to physical activity for those with physical disabilities.

The literature on social support in physical activity settings has demonstrated that encouragement, information, and tangible help from others can positively impact physical activity-related behavior, cognitions and affect. Another social influence can develop within the exercise group itself – cohesion.

Cohesion in Exercise

Cohesion Defined

Group cohesion is a multidimensional construct that is reflected by the group remaining united in attempting to reach its goals and/or for member needs (Carron, Brawley, and Widmeyer, 1998). It is dynamic (i.e., changes over time), and is influenced by multiple factors. Cohesion can be characterized by an individual's attraction to a group or to feelings that the group is a single entity (Carron et al., 1998). Further, these beliefs can be related to the group's task or to social aspects (Carron et al., 1998).

Cohesion and Exercise Adherence

Across a wide variety of settings and samples, cohesion is positively related to exercise adherence. In the first study to examine the cohesion-adherence relationship in exercise, Carron, Widmeyer, and Brawley (1988) compared fitness class participants who had dropped out of university group exercise classes before program completion to those who completed it (i.e., adherers). They found that adherers reported higher task and social cohesion than dropouts, although they examined only one indicator of adherence.

In a similar sample, Spink and Carron (1992) examined the relationship between cohesion and adherence, as assessed by lateness and attendance during the last 4 weeks of a 12-week program. Individuals who were absent and/or late less often reported higher levels of task and social cohesion in the last week of the program. One limitation to these studies was that cohesion was assessed retrospectively – that is, participants were asked about cohesion after the group had ended. Further, only participants attending classes at a university were examined.

To overcome these limitations, Spink and Carron (1994) conducted two studies that assessed cohesion prospectively; cohesion was assessed early in the exercise program while adherence was assessed near program end. In classes from a university setting and from a private fitness club, adherers reported higher levels of task and social cohesion compared to dropouts. This positive cohesion-adherence relationship has been shown to extend to other samples, including older adults (Estabrooks and Carron, 1999a).

Fraser and Spink (2002) examined whether cohesion was related to exercise compliance, the term used to describe adherence to exercise prescribed by health care professionals for prevention or treatment of chronic illness. For example, for an individual prescribed a cardiac rehabilitation program by a doctor, sticking to this program would be termed compliance. These authors found that in a group of patients in a clinical exercise program, higher perceptions of task cohesion were associated with better attendance rates.

Other Outcomes of Cohesion

In addition to examining adherence, researchers have also investigated whether cohesion is related to psychological outcomes. Two studies have specifically examined whether cohesion is related to more positive attitudes to exercise. In a sample of participants attending university fitness classes, Courneya and McAuley (1995) found that task and social cohesion were positively related to attitudes towards exercise. Estabrooks and Carron (1999b) found a similar positive relationship between cohesion and attitude in a sample of older adults. In both samples, attitudes served to mediate the higher adherence rates – that is, cohesion led to more positive attitudes to exercise, which in turn led to better adherence. In older adults, higher perceptions of cohesion are also associated with greater perceptions of control over exercise, as assessed through scheduling self-efficacy (Estabrooks and Carron, 2000). Finally,

Courneya (1995) reported that cohesion (assessed early in the exercise program) was associated with positive affect in university fitness classes.

Teambuilding to Enhance Perceptions of Cohesion

Researchers have investigated whether experimentally increasing perceptions of cohesion through teambuilding can improve these outcomes. Teambuilding refers to any attempt to increase the unity of a group and increase perceptions of cohesion (Carron, Spink, and Prapavessis, 1997). In exercise settings, numerous strategies have been implemented to increase cohesion in an exercise class, including making the group feel distinct, creating group norms, and fostering interaction and communication.

Several studies have implemented a team-building approach to determine its outcomes. For example, Spink and Carron (1993) randomly assigned university fitness classes to either a teambuilding or control condition. They found that rates of dropout and lateness were lower in the classes in which teambuilding was used. Teambuilding groups also reported higher perceptions of control over their exercise. Using a similar design, Carron and Spink (1993) found teambuilding was associated with higher levels of satisfaction in exercisers. Positive effects of teambuilding on adherence and psychological outcomes have also been shown in other samples, including members of private fitness facilities (Annesi, 1999) older adults (Estabrooks and Carron, 1999a), seniors over 80 years old (Watson, Martin Ginis, and Spink, 2006), and cancer patients undergoing chemotherapy (Midtgaard, Rorth, Stelter, and Adamsen, 2006).

Together, this body of literature supports the importance of perceptions of being part of a group in exercise across different settings and populations. It highlights the numerous behavioral, cognitive, and affective outcomes that result from cohesion, and supports the notion that cohesion can be developed in an exercise group through the process of teambuilding. However, in exercise groups, cohesion is not the only social factor related to exercise behaviors, cognitions, and affect. The next section addresses other factors that may be relevant.

Group-Related Factors in Exercise

Exercise Leaders

Exercise leaders can be a powerful social factor in an exercise context. When describing variables that influence dropout behavior from physical activity, Franklin (1986) stated that "although numerous variables affect participant exercise compliance, perhaps the most important is the exercise leader" (p. 12). Two specific types of exercise leaders are group fitness instructors and personal trainers.

Group Fitness Instructors

Group fitness instructors may be a particularly important source of social influence as a single bout of exercise in a group fitness class can have a positive impact on affective outcomes (Lamarche and Gammage, 2010). The leader-exerciser interaction may be particularly significant for individuals initiating exercise (Beauchamp, Welch, and Hulley, 2007; Bray, Gyurcsik, Culos-Reed, Dawson, and Martin, 2001). Bray et al. (2001) examined female participants' confidence in the exercise leader to teach, communicate, and motivate, termed proxy efficacy perceptions. After controlling for self-efficacy, proxy efficacy predicted exercise class attendance in a 10-week fitness program for only those participants with no prior experience of exercise in a structured group class (e.g., exercise initiates). This finding highlights the significant influence an effective exercise leader has on new exercisers' behavior.

We have identified several characteristics of the group fitness instructor that have been shown to positively influence outcomes of exercise participation in group exercise settings. These factors include leadership style, experience and training, and physical characteristics.

Leadership Style

The instructor's enthusiasm, feedback, and ability to motivate have all been used to represent leadership style, which may be one of the most modifiable and relevant characteristics of the group fitness instructor. In male and female fitness class participants, Evans, Cotter, and Roy (2005) found that enthusiasm or motivation was the most important characteristic of fitness instructors. Qualitative research has also provided evidence of the importance of leadership style in a group exercise setting (Bain, Wilson, and Chaikind, 1989; Estabrooks et al., 2004; Fox et al., 2007). Participants report that it is important for the leader to have a warm, caring and compassionate personality toward class members, and that a welcoming versus unfriendly instructor positively impacts class attendance (Fox et al., 2007).

Quantitative research has compared the effects of an enriched versus bland leadership style (Turner, Rejeski, and Brawley, 1997). An enriched leadership style is characterized by frequent technical instruction and support, positive skill-related feedback and encouragement, the use of class participants' names, individual attention, and general conversation before and after the class. By contrast, a bland leadership style is created by omitting support, encouragement and social interaction between the leader and class participants, vague, group-directed feedback, and negatively-worded corrections to technique. Research has shown that female participants led by an instructor using an enriched leadership style report greater increases in self-efficacy and positive affect (revitalization) than participants led by an instructor using a bland leadership style (Turner et al., 1997). Subsequent studies have provided additional empirical support for the positive impact of an enriched leadership style in group exercise classes (Bray, Millen, Eidsness, and Leuzinger, 2005; Fox, Rejeski, and Gauvin, 2000; Martin and Fox, 2001).

Other leadership styles have also been compared. In a sample of female participants with high social physique anxiety, Raedeke, Focht, and Scales (2007) found that participants led by a leader using a health-oriented leadership style reported more positive affect, less exhaustion, and stronger future intentions to join a similar group exercise class than women led by a leader using an appearance-oriented leadership style.

The research findings described thus far under leadership style have examined the impact of leadership style in one single exercise session; leadership style has also been examined across a longitudinal exercise program (Beauchamp, Welch et al., 2007; Edmunds, Ntoumanis, and Duda, 2008). For example, Edmunds et al. (2008) investigated the impact of a self-determination theory-based teaching style (versus a typical teaching style) on affect, psychological need satisfaction, motivational regulations, behavioral intention, and class attendance over a 10-week exercise program. Participants led by the instructor using the self-determination theory-based teaching style showed a greater increase in relatedness and competence need satisfaction, more positive affect, and higher attendance rates than the control group.

Experience and Training

Experience and training are also important characteristics of group fitness instructors. For example, being able to cue and show proper technique, being able to lead a variety of activities, and being certified were commonly cited as important characteristics of fitness leaders (Evans et al., 2005). In addition, having highly qualified fitness instructors was among the top reasons for women's choice of fitness club (Szumilewicz, 2011).

There is qualitative support that the exercise leader's experience and training can positively impact exercisers' experiences (Estabrooks et al., 2004; Fox et al., 2007). Estabrooks et al. (2004) explored perceptions of leadership in physical activity groups of older adults. Participants described characteristics such as being qualified, knowledgeable, having certification, and possessing good presentation skills as important qualities of group leaders in physical activity. These findings are consistent with Fox et al. (2007) who found that leadership expertise was described by participants as important, particularly in the beginning stages of a program, which was the most difficult time.

Physical Characteristics of the Exercise Leader

Although perhaps relatively less important than leadership style or experience, research examining the influence of physical characteristics (e.g., body shape and size, sex, race, or age; Evans et al., 2005) of the exercise leader on exercise-related outcomes should be mentioned.

Physical Fitness

One physical aspect of the leader that has been mentioned by class participants as important is physical fitness. Participants have reported that the exercise leader must "look the part" (Estabrooks et al., 2004, p. 240) and "be in good shape themselves" (Estabrooks et al., 2004, p. 240) in order for participants to look up to the instructor as a role model. Evans et al. (2005) found that being physically fit was the second most reported characteristic of the exercise leader to be deemed important.

Leader Gender

In an imagined exercise class, Bray, Bassett, and Amirthavasar (2011) examined self-monitoring as a potential moderator of self-presentational concerns in same-sex or co-ed group exercise settings in women. The findings showed that high self-monitors reported lower social physique anxiety after imagining exercising in a male-led group exercise class.

In an actual group exercise class, Lamarche and Gammage (2010) manipulated gender of the group exercise leader to examine its impact. These authors found no influence of exercise instructor gender on self-presentational efficacy, state social anxiety or social physique anxiety following the exercise class. In fact, all variables improved following the class, regardless of instructor gender.

Physique Salience

A third physical characteristic that has received some investigation is the physique salience of the group fitness instructor (Crawford and Eklund, 1994; Eklund and Crawford, 1994; Fleming and Martin Ginis, 2004; Martin Ginis, Prapavessis, and Haase, 2008; Sinden, Martin Ginis, and Angove, 2003). Physique salience is typically manipulated by changing the level of emphasis on the body's appearance through exercise clothing (i.e., shorts and a loose fitting t-shirt versus spandex shorts and a jog bra). Although researchers have hypothesized that leaders wearing clothing that emphasizes the body's appearance would elicit self-presentational concerns, which in turn, would lead to negative exercise-related outcomes and prevent individuals from experiencing the positive benefits of group exercise, findings have generally not supported this hypothesis. Instead, these studies show that examining other variables such as physical activity level, trait social physique anxiety, and direction of social comparisons to the leader may be important moderators that influence reactions to group exercise class in general (Crawford and Eklund, 1994; Martin Ginis et al., 2008; Sinden et al., 2003).

Personal Trainers

The second type of exercise leader that can have a powerful source of social influence in an exercise setting is personal trainers.

The Presence of Personal Trainers

Jackson (2010) argued that personal trainers can have a positive influence on self-efficacy, which can in turn increase adherence to exercise. Personal trainers may be particularly effective for novice exercisers who may not know how to develop an exercise program to reach personal goals or how to perform exercises correctly.

Clients have described the positive outcomes associated with using personal trainers (Madeson, Hultquist, Church, and Fisher, 2010; Melton, Dail, Katula, and Mustian, 2011). In qualitative studies, personal training was described as a positive experience including "enjoyable, fun and meaningful" (Madeson et al., 2010, p. 160). Motivation also emerged as a main theme and was described in terms of feeling accountable to their personal trainer. Motivation served as a factor in their adherence to exercise such that participants felt accountable to go to the gym, keep their personal training appointment, and to work hard for their trainer. Motivation in the form of encouragement was also noted – personal trainers provided inspiration by exercising with them, and being a fit and healthy role model.

Fischer and Bryant (2008) and McClaran (2003) examined the impact of personal trainers on movement through the stages of the transtheoretical model. McClaran (2003) found significant upward movement through the stages at program end. Fischer and Bryant (2008) compared the effectiveness of a personal trainer on exercisers to matched participants not using personal training services. Their results compliment those of McClaran (2003) – control participants showed a significant regression in stage of change scores and a decrease in cognitive and behavioral processes of change, decisional balance, and scheduling self-efficacy. A greater number of participants classified as active maintainers or progressors were found in the personal trainer group compared to the control group. Because the majority of participants in both groups were categorized in the maintenance stage at baseline, these findings may provide support for the effectiveness of a personal trainer on exercise initiation.

The effectiveness of personal trainers has also been demonstrated in a sample of outpatients who were obese. Jeffery, Wing, Thorson, and Burton (1998) compared five treatment groups on adherence and weight loss. All participants received standard behavior therapy, with the other treatment conditions adding supervised walks, supervised walks with a personal trainer, supervised walks and financial incentive, and supervised walks with a personal trainer and financial incentive. After the 12-month program, a personal trainer and financial incentive led to the highest adherence, and when used together, the number of walks attended was three times as high as supervised walks only.

Characteristics of Effective Personal Trainers

Researchers have also provided insight into the qualities of personal trainers that are important for a client to have a positive experience with personal training support (Madeson et al., 2010; Melton et al., 2011). Specifically, being optimistic and fun, having skills that maximized client effort, understanding of clients' capabilities and limits, having competence in designing workouts and teaching technique, and fostering personal friendship were deemed important to their experience with their personal trainer. Being able to develop an effective program in which participants noticed physical and psychological improvements (i.e., weight loss, strength, and functionality, self-confidence, feeling better, and having more energy) was also reported as being important to their personal training experience. Gender was also identified as an important trainer quality for some female participants, as they believed a female trainer would have a better understanding of women's bodies.

Co-Exercisers

Another significant source of social influence in a group exercise setting is the co-exercisers, who may be a powerful source of social support for continued participation and enjoyment.

Perceived Similarity of Co-Exercisers

Perceived similarity is an important quality of the exercise group that positively impacts exercise-related outcomes. For example, Bain et al. (1989) examined perceptions of exercise programs in a sample of people who were obese. Participants indicated a preference to exercise in a group of people who were also obese because they felt they had a shared experience of perceived social disapproval based on weight status. Further, exercising with like others based on weight increased their motivation and comfort level.

Quantitative research has begun to describe the preference of exercising with similar others. This area of research has examined two general types of similarity: surface- and deep-level similarity. Surface-level similarity is defined as overt characteristics that are typically physical in nature (i.e., age, gender, weight status, physical condition and appearance), while deep-level similarity is defined as qualities that are not overtly observable and oftentimes discovered through extended interaction (e.g., attitudes, beliefs, values; Harrison, Price, and Bell, 1998).

One study examined exercise preferences of participants (30 to 91 years of age) for involvement in standard exercise classes (Beauchamp, Carron et al., 2007). Individuals had a preference for exercising with others of a similar age and participants rated such contexts relatively more appealing than those involving co-exercisers of considerable age differences. Dunlop and Beauchamp (2011b) found that male and female participants reported a stronger preference to exercise in a gender-segregated versus gender-integrated group exercise environment. Further, weight status was shown to moderate this relationship; individuals who were overweight versus normal weight reported a stronger relative preference for gender-segregated group exercise contexts.

Beyond preferences for exercise, recent research has examined outcomes such as class attendance and cohesion (Beauchamp, Dunlop, Downy, and Estabrooks, 2012; Dunlop and Beauchamp, 2011a). Dunlop and Beauchamp (2011a) examined the relationship between perceived similarity and cohesion (task and social cohesion). Perceived deep-level similarity predicted task cohesion while surface-level cohesion predicted social cohesion following the 8th class of the program. Further, perceived surface-level, but not deep-level, similarity prospectively predicted attendance at the 8th class session. Findings from a study examining perceived surface- and deep-level similarity in members of a postnatal exercise class also show support for perceived similarity (Beauchamp et al., 2012). Specifically, perceptions of surface-level similarity, particularly with respect to class members' age, predicted class attendance of a postnatal exercise class.

Group Atmosphere

Similar to the manipulation of leadership style, two types of group atmospheres have been compared: enriched versus bland. In the enriched group condition, confederates are used to foster social interaction in a comfortable and relaxed setting. Specifically, confederates introduce themselves to other participants, engage in casual conversation, and verbally make encouraging and positive remarks to the leader and to the class as a whole. In the bland group environment condition, confederates avoid social interaction with other class participants and the exercise leader, to create a neutral, non-interactive environment.

In an experimental design, Fox et al. (2000) examined the impact of the group environment (in addition to leadership style) during a single group exercise class in novice exercisers on enjoyment and likelihood of joining a similar class in the future. Findings showed that participants in the enriched condition reported higher enjoyment and intentions to join a similar class in the future than the bland condition. These findings suggest the added benefit of an enriched group environment on enjoyment and future intentions for novice exercisers.

In a related study, Martin and Fox (2001) examined the impact of the group environment (in addition to leadership style) on social anxiety in a single group exercise class. Their results revealed that participants in the bland condition reported less social anxiety than those in the enriched condition. This finding is particularly interesting given that participants in the bland condition rated the group atmosphere as less positive than those in the enriched condition – a finding consistent with Fox et al. (2000). Martin and Fox (2001) suggested that a lack of social interaction between group members may have led participants to feel more anonymous, thus reducing worries about others' evaluations (i.e., social anxiety). These findings suggest that for new exercisers, an enriched group environment may lead to greater enjoyment and increase the probability of future participation (Fox et al., 2000), but may also increase social anxiety (Martin and Fox, 2001). However, it appears that an enriched leader may help participants override their worry about others' evaluations (Fox et al., 2000; Martin and Fox, 2001).

Group Size

Another factor that has been associated with exercise-related outcomes in groups is group size. Carron, Brawley, and Widmeyer (1990) noted that there may be benefits of exercising in large groups due to increased opportunity to meet desirable others. For example in an exercise class, large groups may offer the opportunity to meet more individuals with whom one has common interests, or it may allow people to feel that they can 'blend in with the crowd', rather than being the center of attention. On the other hand, increasing group size may also have negative outcomes. For instance, large groups may mean less personal attention from the instructor or fewer resources such as space or equipment.

Group Size and Adherence

Two studies have investigated whether smaller or larger class sizes are associated with better adherence. Remers, Widmeyer, Williams, and Meyers (1995) investigated medium (18-26 participants) and large (70-90 participants) sized exercise classes and found that attendance was better in larger classes. In a wider range of class sizes, Carron et al. (1990) investigated attendance and dropout in 4 different class sizes in a university setting: small (12-17 participants), medium (18-26 participants) moderately large (27-31 participants) and large (32-46 participants). They found a curvilinear relationship between adherence and class size. Attendance was significantly higher and dropout was significantly lower in the small and large class sizes compared to the other two sizes. Interestingly, there was no difference in adherence between the small and large classes.

Group Size and Perceptions of Cohesion

Remers et al. (1995) also investigated whether perceptions of cohesion differed between medium and large classes. They found that cohesion was higher in the large classes. Using a slightly different definition of class size (small classes fewer than 20 participants and large classes more than 40 participants), Carron and Spink (1995) found that in week 3, the small classes had higher task cohesion than the large classes. However, after week 8, small classes had higher perceptions of both task and social cohesion. Further, perceptions of cohesion increased across time in the small groups, but decreased over time in the large groups. However, Carron and Spink (1995) found a teambuilding intervention was equally effective at increasing perceptions of cohesion in small and large classes.

Group Size and Cognitive and Affective Outcomes

Remers et al. (1995) investigated other outcomes related to class size in medium and large exercise classes. They found that members of large classes perceived that they exerted themselves at optimal levels more frequently than members of medium classes, were more satisfied in their classes, and had a more positive perception of their classes. Carron et al. (1990) examined a variety of outcomes in three different exercise class sizes at a university: small (6-13 participants), medium (25-39 participants), and large (more than 75 participants). Each group met 3 times per week for 10-12 weeks during the semester. Small classes were associated with the most positive perceptions of the instructor; perceptions of the instructor decreased as the class size increased. With respect to opportunities for interaction, perceptions increased from small to medium classes, but then decreased from medium to large classes. Further, participants in large classes perceived more crowding than either of the other classes. Finally, satisfaction with classes decreased from small to medium and again from medium to large classes. However, it should be noted that although larger groups were generally perceived more negatively across a variety of outcomes, the magnitude of the differences was relatively small, suggesting that it is possible to provide positive experiences even in large exercise classes.

PRACTICAL IMPLICATIONS

Based on the previous review of the literature on social factors in exercise settings, we have provided the following recommendations to allow practitioners to use social influences to increase exercise behavior and provide positive psychological experiences across a variety of settings and samples.

Increasing Social Support

Evidence clearly shows social support can increase exercise behavior – thus it is important to provide multiple types of social support from multiple sources. How can social support be provided to most effectively increase exercise behavior?

1) Social support should attempt to increase feelings of self-efficacy. For example, friends can provide verbal persuasion to increase confidence that exercise can be scheduled into one's life, even in challenging times. Professionals can be very important as well. For instance, providing instructions or directions on how much to exercise, what kind of exercise to do, or how to perform specific exercises to clients or patients may help to increase their confidence to be able to actually perform these activities, which is essential for their performance.
2) Ask family and friends to help provide social support – this could be in the form of reminding people to exercise, encouraging them to keep working hard, or providing assistance – helping with errands to free up time to exercise for example.
3) Finding an exercise buddy can also increase exercise behavior – this can help people feel motivated and encouraged towards their exercise. It also provides a role model

for exercise. Along similar lines, family and friends should be sure to watch others be active even if they are not active themselves – particularly for children and adolescents.

4) In some cases, it is possible that social support may be harmful – for example, if people feel that they are being controlled or someone is telling them what to do, they may respond by doing the opposite – not exercising. Thus, it is important that social support be delivered effectively – it should be believable and positive.

Increasing Cohesion

The process of teambuilding is ongoing. The following recommendations provide some examples of how teambuilding can be implemented – but no two exercise groups are alike – what works for one group may not be effective for another.

1) Teambuilding effectively consists of several specific stages, which include: the introductory stage, in which the link between cohesion and positive outcomes are discussed with the fitness leader; the conceptual stage, in which factors that can impact cohesion in an exercise group are described; the practical stage, in which ideas to increase cohesion in a group are generated; and the intervention stage, in which those ideas are implemented by the group leader (Carron et al., 1997).
2) Several specific teambuilding elements have been utilized previously to increase cohesion. For example, interaction and communication between group members can be increased by using partner work. The group can be made more distinct by having a special name or a group t-shirt. Setting group goals helps foster cohesion by encouraging people to work together. Social cohesion can be fostered by group members getting together outside of the exercise class – maybe for coffee. Developing specific roles and norms within the group is important. Group members may agree to always stay for the entire class no matter how busy they feel. More experienced group members may take on a leadership role within the group. Finally, sacrifice can help increase cohesion – perhaps making the workout easier for one day if someone is not feeling well.

Creating Positive Group Exercise Environments

Generally, group fitness instructors and personal trainers can have a positive influence on exercise-related outcomes, particularly for those initiating exercise. The specific strategies used will vary from group to group based on member characteristics and preferences.

1) Probably the most important characteristics of fitness leaders are those related to leadership style versus physical characteristics. Fitness leaders need to consciously incorporate strategies that foster positive social interaction. Some specific practical suggestions for developing an enriched leadership style include using class participants' names, providing specific individualized instruction, providing attention and positive reinforcement to each class member, engaging in general conversation

before and after the class, and rewarding the effort of the class. Personal trainers should also foster positive social interaction. The same principles described above that have been used by group fitness instructors can also be applied in personal training settings.

2) Fitness facilities as well as individual instructors and trainers should be sure to make their qualifications known up front to their clients to help establish their expertise and build confidence in them from their clients.
3) Create fitness programs made up of people who are similar to one another – especially for those who may be apprehensive about exercise (e.g., beginners, seniors, overweight/obese individuals, those with chronic conditions, women). By matching groups on these factors, individuals may feel more confident and less self-conscious, and may have a more positive experience overall. Similarity amongst group members may also help to foster cohesion.
4) Any group size can be effective, but an exercise program must be tailored to the size. In bigger groups, instructors must find way to provide feedback and attention to everyone – maybe by moving around the class and providing feedback or by learning participants' names. In small groups, instructors must be aware not to draw too much attention to people as it may make them self-conscious. By managing expectations of participants ahead of time, participants in any group size can have a positive experience.

KEY POINTS

In this final section, we present our thoughts on the importance of social influences in physical activity settings. These points relate to both research and practice.

1) With respect to social support, the literature is extremely inconsistent in how it measures and defines both the type and sources of social support. It is thus difficult to compare findings across studies, and perhaps accounts for some of the conflicting findings. For example, where studies may not find evidence that social support impacts physical activity behavior, it could be due to the fact that the relevant type or source was not assessed. Researchers must work to address this limitation in the future.
2) Related to this point above, qualitative studies seem to show much more robust effects of social support on a variety of outcomes, both psychological and physical. These findings should not be underestimated – again, they may reflect the fact that there is a real challenge in quantifying social support for exercise.
3) With respect to examining how social influences impact exercise, the greatest diversity has been in the social support research. However, even our understanding of social support comes primarily from healthy populations. We are only just beginning to understand how special populations (e.g., chronic disease, disability) may benefit from social support. Future research should continue to expand the populations that are investigated.

4) Related to cohesion and creating positive group environments, the research has primarily been limited to structured group exercise classes with female exercisers – and often investigates only 'traditional' types of exercise such as aerobics. However, given that many people do not like to exercise in structured settings, it is imperative that we begin to understand how to implement teambuilding and positive exercise environments into less structured settings. Further, given the rise of activities such as mind-body (e.g., yoga, Pilates) and more 'back-to-basics' approaches (e.g., boot camp, Crossfit, calisthenics), we need to examine how social influence may be important in these types of exercise.
5) For personal trainers and fitness instructors, knowledge and credibility are critical influences. Currently, there are a wide variety of certifying bodies with differing requirements. Some standardization across these organizations is imperative so people know what they are getting from professionals. More importantly, these organizations need to address social influences in their training programs so personal trainers and fitness instructors provide the best possible experiences for their clients.
6) Social media (e.g., Twitter, Facebook, Pinterest) may offer an entirely new way of providing social influence. Research must address how influential these platforms are, how to use them most effectively, and how to target those most in need. It is possible that through social media, we can provide social support even in those who prefer to exercise alone, who are self-conscious about exercising with others, or who are hard to reach.

REFERENCES

Alcock, J. E., Carment, D. W., and Sadava, S. W. (1991). *A textbook of social psychology* (2nd ed.). Scarborough, ON: Prentice Hall.

Anderson, E. S., Wojcik, J. R., Winett, R. A., and Williams, D. M. (2006). Social-cognitive determinants of physical activity: The influence of social support, self-efficacy, outcome expectations, and self-regulation among participants in a church-based health promotion study. *Health Psychology, 25*, 510-520.

Annesi, J. J. (1999). Effects of minimal group promotion on cohesion and exercise adherence. *Small Group Research, 30*, 542-557.

Ayotte, B. J., Margrett, J. A., and Hicks-Patrick, J. (2010). Physical activity in middle-aged and young-old adults: The roles of self-efficacy, barriers, outcome expectancies, self-regulatory behaviors and social support. *Journal of Health Psychology, 15*, 173-185.

Bain, L. L., Wilson, T., and Chaikind, E. (1989). Participant perception of exercise programs for overweight women. *Research Quarterly for Exercise and Sport, 60*, 134-143.

Balde, A., Figueras, J., Hawkins, D. A., and Miller, J. R. (2003). Physician advice to the elderly about physical activity. *Journal of Aging and Physical Activity, 11*, 90-97.

Bandura, A. (1997). *Self-efficacy: The exercise of control.* New York, NY: W. H. Freeman.

Bandura, A. (2005). The primacy of self-regulation in health promotion. *Applied Psychology, 54*, 245-254.

Bauman, A. E., Reis, R. S., Sallis, J. F., Wells, J. C., Loos, R. J. F., and Martin, B. W. (2012). Correlates of physical activity: Why are some people physically active and others not? *Lancet, 380*, 258-271.

Beauchamp, M. R., Carron, B. V., McCutcheon, S., and Harper, O. (2007). Older adults' preferences for exercising along versus in groups: Considering contextual congruence. *Annals of Behavioral Medicine, 33*, 200-206.

Beauchamp, M. R., Dunlop, W. L., Downey, S. M., and Estabrooks, P. A. (2012). First impressions count: Perceptions of surface-level and deep-level similarity within postnatal exercise classes and implications for program adherence. *Journal of Health Psychology, 17*, 68-76.

Beauchamp, M. R., Welch, A. S., and Hulley, A. J. (2007). Transformational and transactional leadership and exercise-related self-efficacy: An exploratory study. *Journal of Health Psychology, 12*, 83-88.

Beets, M. W., Cardinal, B. J., and Alderman, B. L. (2010). Parental social support and the physical activity-related behaviors of youth: A review. *Health Education and Behavior, 37*, 621-644.

Beets, M. W., Pitetti, K. H., and Forlaw, L. (2007). The role of self-efficacy and referent specific social support in promoting rural adolescent girls' physical activity. *American Journal of Health Behavior, 31*, 227-237.

Bray, S. R., Bassett, R. L., and Amirthavasar, G. (2011). Self-monitoring and women's self-presentational reactions to variations in sex of the exercise class instructor and co-exercisers. *Journal of Applied Biobehavioral Research, 16*, 1-15.

Bray, S. R., Gyurcsik, N. C., Culos-Reed, S. N., Dawson, K. A., and Martin, K. A. (2001). An exploratory investigation of the relationship between proxy efficacy, self-efficacy and exercise attendance. *Journal of Health Psychology, 6*, 425-434.

Bray, S. R., Millen, J. A., Eidsness, J., and Leuzinger, C. (2005). The effects of leadership style and exercise program choreography on enjoyment and intentions to exercise. *Psychology of Sport and Exercise, 6*, 415-425.

Burke, S. M., Carron, A. V., and Eys, M. A. (2006). Physical activity context: Preferences of university students. *Psychology of Sport and Exercise, 7*, 1-13.

Burke, S. M., Carron, A. V., Eys, M. A., Ntoumanis, N., and Estabrooks, P. A. (2006). Group versus individual approach? A meta-analysis of the effectiveness of interventions to promote physical activity. *Sport and Exercise Psychology Review, 2*, 19-35.

Burke, S. M., Carron, A. V., and Shapcott, K. M. (2008). Cohesion in exercise groups: An overview. *International Journal of Sport and Exercise Psychology, 1*, 107-123.

Carron, A. V., Brawley, L. R., and Widmeyer, W. N. (1990). The impact of group size in an exercise setting. *Journal of Sport and Exercise Psychology, 12*, 376-387.

Carron, A. V., Brawley, L. R., and Widmeyer, W. N. (1998). The measurement of cohesiveness in sport groups. In J. L. Duda (Ed.), *Advances in sport and exercise psychology measurement* (pp. 213-226). Morgantown, WV: Fitness Information Technology.

Carron, A. V., Hausenblas, H. A., and Mack, D. (1996). Social influence and exercise: A meta-analysis. *Journal of Sport and Exercise Psychology, 18*, 1-16.

Carron, A. V., and Spink, K. S. (1993). Team building in an exercise setting. *The Sport Psychologist, 7*, 8-18.

Carron, A. V., and Spink, K. S. (1995). The group size-cohesion relationship in minimal groups. *Small Group Research, 26*, 86-105.

Carron, A. V., Spink, K. S., and Prapavessis, H. (1997). Team building and cohesiveness in the sport and exercise setting: Use of indirect interventions. *Journal of Applied Sport Psychology, 9*, 61-72.

Carron, A. V., Widmeyer, W. N., and Brawley, L. R. (1988). Group cohesion and individual adherence to physical activity. *Journal of Sport and Exercise Psychology, 10*, 127-138.

Clark, D., Patrick, D., and Grembowski, D. (1995). Socioeconomic status and exercise self-efficacy in late life. *Journal of Behavioral Medicine, 18*, 355-375.

Courneya, K. S. (1995). Cohesion correlates with affect in structured exercise classes. *Perceptual and Motor Skills, 81*, 1021-1022.

Courneya, K. S., and McAuley, E. (1995). Cognitive mediators of the social influence-exercise adherence relationship: A test of the theory of planned behavior. *Journal of Behavioral Medicine, 18*, 499-515.

Crawford, S., and Eklund, R. C. (1994). Social physique anxiety, reasons for exercise, and attitudes toward exercise settings. *Journal of Sport and Exercise Psychology, 16*, 70-82.

Dracup, K. (1994). Cardiac rehabilitation: The role of social support in recovery and compliance. In S. A. Shumaker, and S. M. Czajkowski (Eds.), *Social support and cardiovascular disease* (pp. 333-353). New York, NY: Plenum Press.

Duncan, S. C. (1993). The role of cognitive appraisal and friendship provisions in adolescents' affect and motivation toward activity in physical education. *Research Quarterly for Exercise and Sport, 64*, 314.

Duncan, S. C., Duncan, T. E., and Strycker, L. A. (2005). Sources and types of social support in youth physical activity. *Health Psychology, 24*, 3-10.

Duncan, T. E., and McAuley, E. (1993). Social support and efficacy cognitions in exercise adherence: A latent growth curve analysis. *Journal of Behavioral Medicine, 16*, 199-218.

Dunlop, W. L., and Beauchamp, M. R. (2011a). Does similarity make a difference? Predicting cohesion and attendance behaviors within exercise group settings. *Group Dynamics: Theory, Research, and Practice, 15*, 258-266.

Dunlop, W. L., and Beauchamp, M. R. (2011b). En-gendering choice: Preferences for exercising in gender-segregated and gender-integrated groups and consideration of overweight status. *International Journal of Behavioral Medicine, 18*, 216-220.

Edmunds, J., Ntoumanis, N., and Duda, J. L. (2008). Testing a self-determination theory-based teaching style intervention in the exercise domain. *European Journal of Social Psychology, 38*, 375-388.

Eklund, R. C., and Crawford, S. (1994). Active women, social physique anxiety, and exercise. *Journal of Sport and Exercise Psychology, 16*, 431-448.

Erling, J., and Oldridge, N. B. (1985). Effects of a spousal-support program on compliance with cardiac rehabilitation. *Medicine in Science Sports and Exercise, 17*, 284.

Estabrooks, P. A., and Carron, A. V. (1999a). Group cohesion in older adult exercisers: Prediction and intervention effects. *Journal of Behavioral Medicine, 22*, 575-588.

Estabrooks, P. A., and Carron, A.V. (1999b). The influence of the group with elderly exercisers. *Small Group Research, 30,* 438-452.

Estabrooks, P. A., and Carron, A. V. (2000). Predicting scheduling self-efficacy in older adult exercisers: The role of task cohesion. *Journal of Aging and Physical Activity, 8,* 41-50.

Estabrooks, P. A., Munroe, K. J., Fox, E. H., Gyurcsik, N. C., Hill, J. L., Lyon, R., Rosenkranz, S., and Shannon, V. R. (2004). Leadership in physical activity groups for older adults: A qualitative analysis. *Journal of Aging and Physical Activity, 12*, 232-245.

Evans, R. R., Cotter, E. M., and Roy, J. L. (2005). Preferred body type of fitness instructors among university students in exercise classes. *Perceptual and Motor Skills, 101*, 257-266.

Eyler, A., Brownson, R., Donatelle, R., King, A., Brown, D., and Sallis, J. (1999). Physical activity social support and middle-and older-aged minority women: Results from a U.S. survey. *Social Science and Medicine, 49*, 781-789.

Fischer, D. V., and Bryant, J. (2008). Effect of certified personal trainer services on stage of exercise behavior and exercise mediators in female college students. *Journal of American College Health, 56*, 369-376.

Fleming, J. C., and Martin Ginis, K. A. (2004). The effects of commercial exercise video models on women's self-presentational efficacy and exercise task self-efficacy. *Journal of Applied Sport Psychology, 16*, 92-102.

Fox, K. R., Stathi, A., McKenna, J., and Davis, M. G. (2007). Physical activity and mental well-being in older people participating in the Better Ageing Project. *European Journal of Applied Physiology, 100*, 591-602.

Fox, L. D., Rejeski, W. J., and Gauvin, L. (2000). Effects of leadership style and group dynamics on enjoyment of physical activity. *American Journal of Health Promotion, 14*, 277-283.

Franklin, B. A. (1986). Clinical components of a successful adults fitness program. *American Journal of Health Promotion, 1*, 6-13.

Franklin, B. A. (1988). Program factors that influence exercise adherence: Practical adherence skills for the clinical staff. In R. K. Dishman (Ed.), *Exercise adherence: Its impact on public health* (pp. 237-258). Champaign, IL: Human Kinetics.

Fraser, S. N., and Rodgers, W. M. (2012). The influence of general and exercise specific social support on self-efficacy for overcoming barriers to cardiac rehabilitation. *Journal of Applied Social Psychology, 42*, 1811-1829.

Fraser, S. N., and Spink, K. S. (2002). Examining the role of social support and group cohesion in exercise compliance. *Journal of Behavioral Medicine, 25*, 233-249.

Gottlieb, B. H., and Bergen, A. E. (2010). Social support concepts and measures. *Journal of Psychosomatic Research, 69*, 511-520.

Harrison, D. A., Price, K. H., and Bell, M. P. (1998). Beyond relational demography: Time and the effect of surface- and deep-level diversity on work group cohesion. *Academy of Management Journal, 41*, 96–107.

Helgeson, V. S., and Cohen, S. (1996). Social support and adjustment to cancer: Reconciling descriptive, correlational, and intervention research. *Health Psychology, 15*, 135-148.

Hohepa, M., Scragg, R., Schofield, G., Kolt, G. S., and Schaaf, D. (2007). Social support for youth physical activity: Importance of siblings, parents, friends and school support across a segmented school day. *International Journal of Behavioral Nutrition and Physical Activity, 4*, 54.

Jackson, D. (2010). How personal trainers can use self-efficacy theory to enhance exercise behavior in beginning exercisers. *Strength and Conditioning Journal, 32*, 67-71.

Jeffery, R. W., Wing, R. R., Thorson, C., and Burton, L. R. (1998). Use of personal trainers and financial incentives to increase exercise in a behavioral weight-loss program. *Journal of Consulting and Clinical Psychology, 66*, 777-783.

Junker, L., and Carlberg, E. B. (2011). Factors that affect exercise participation among people with physical disabilities. *Advances in Physiotherapy, 13*, 18-25.

King, A. C., Castro, C., Wilcox, S., Eyler, A. A., Sallis, J. F., and Brownson, R. C. (2000). Personal and environmental factors associated with physical inactivity among different racial-ethnic groups of U.S. middle-aged and older-aged women. *Health Psychology, 19*, 354-64.

King, A. C., Haskell, W. L., Taylor, C. B., Kraemer, H. C., and DeBusk, R. F. (1991). Group- vs. home-based exercise training in healthy older men and women. *Journal of the American Medical Association, 266*, 1535-1542.

Lamarche, L., and Gammage, K. L. (2010). The effects of leader gender on self-presentational concerns in exercise. *Psychology and Health, 25*, 769-781.

Lehnert, K., Sudeck, G., and Conselmann, A. (2012). Subjective well-being and exercise in the second half of life: A critical review of theoretical approaches. *European Review of Aging and Physical Activity, 9*, 87-102.

Macdonald-Wallis, K., Jago, R., Page, A. S., Brockman, R., and Thompson, J. L. (2011). School-based friendship networks and children's physical activity: A spatial analytical approach. *Social Science and Medicine, 73*, 6-12.

Macdonald-Wallis, K., Jago, R., and Sterne, J. A. C. (2012). Social network analysis of childhood and youth physical activity. *American Journal of Preventive Medicine, 43*, 636-642.

Madeson, M. N., Hultquist, C. N., Church, A., and Fisher, L. A. (2010). A phenomenological investigation of women's experiences with personal training. *International Journal of Exercise Science, 3*, 157-169.

Martin, K. A., and Fox, L. D. (2001). Group and leadership effects on social anxiety experienced during an exercise class. *Journal of Applied Social Psychology, 31*, 1000-1016.

Martin Ginis, K. A., Prapavessis, H., and Haase, A. M. (2008). The effects of physique-salient and physique non-salient exercise videos on women's body image, self-presentational concerns, and exercise motivation. *Body Image, 5*, 164-172.

McAuley, E., Blissmer, B., Marquez, D. X., Jerome, G. J., Kramer, A. F., and Katula, J. (2000). Social relations, physical activity, and well-being in older adults. *Preventive Medicine, 31*, 608-617.

McAuley, E., Elavsky, S., Jerome, G. J., Konopack, J. F., and Marquez, D. X. (2005). Physical activity-related well-being in older adults: Social cognitive influences. *Psychology and Aging, 20*, 295-302.

McClaran, S. R. (2003). The effectiveness of personal training on changing attitudes towards physical activity. *Journal of Sports Science and Medicine, 2*, 10-14.

McDonough, M. H., Sabiston, C. M., and Crocker, P. R. E. (2008). An interpretative phenomenological examination of psychosocial changes among breast cancer survivors in their first season of dragon boating. *Journal of Applied Sport Psychology, 20*, 425-440.

McDonough, M. H., Sabiston, C. M., and Ullrich-French, S. (2011). The development of social relationship, social support, and posttraumatic growth in a dragon boating team for breast cancer survivors. *Journal of Sport and Exercise Psychology, 33*, 627-648.

Melton, D., Dail, T. K., Katula, J. A., and Mustian, K. M. (2011). Women's perspectives of personal trainers: A qualitative study. *The Sport Journal, 14*.

Midtgaard, J., Rorth, M., Stelter, R., and Adamsen, L. (2006). The group matters: An explorative study of group cohesion and quality of life in cancer patients participating in physical exercise intervention during treatment. *European Journal of Cancer Care, 15*, 25-33.

Motl, R. W., Dishman, R. K., Saunders, R. P., Dowda, M., and Pate, R. R. (2007). Perceptions of physical and social environment variables and self-efficacy as correlates of self-reported physical activity among adolescent girls. *Journal of Pediatric Psychology, 32*, 6-12.

Motl, R. W., and McAuley, E. (2009). Pathways between physical activity and quality of life in adults with multiple sclerosis. *Health Psychology, 28*, 682-689.

Motl, R. W., McAuley, E., and Snook, E. M. (2007). Physical activity and quality of life in multiple sclerosis: Possible roles of social support, self-efficacy, and functional limitations. *Rehabilitation Psychology, 52*, 143-151.

Motl, R. W., McAuley, E., Snook, E. M., and Gliottoni, R. C. (2009). Physical activity and quality of life in multiple sclerosis: Intermediary roles of disability, fatigue, mood, pain, self-efficacy and social support. *Psychology, Health and Medicine, 14*, 111-124.

Motl, R. W., Snook, E. M., McAuley, E., Scott, J. A., and Douglass, M. L. (2006). Correlates of physical activity among individuals with multiple sclerosis. *Annals of Behavioral Medicine, 32,* 154-161.

Parry, D. C. (2007). "There is *life* after breast cancer": Nine vignettes exploring dragon boat racing for breast cancer survivors. *Leisure Sciences, 29,* 53-69.

Parry, D. C. (2008). The contribution of dragon boat racing to women's health and breast cancer survivorship. *Qualitative Health Research, 18,* 222-233.

Pridgeon, L., and Grogan, S. (2012). Understanding exercise adherence and dropout: An interpretative phenomenological analysis of men and women's accounts of gym attendance and non-attendance. *Qualitative Research in Sport, Exercise and Health, 4,* 382-399.

Prochaska, J. J., Rodgers, M. W., and Sallis, J. F. (2002). Association of parent and peer support with adolescent physical activity. *Research Quarterly for Exercise and Sport, 73,* 206-210.

Raedeke, T. D., Focht, B. C., and Scales, D. (2007). Social environment factors and psychological responses to acute exercise for socially physique anxious females. *Psychology of Sport and Exercise, 8*, 463-476.

Ravenek, M. J., and Schneider, M. A. (2009). Social support for physical activity and perceptions of control in early Parkinson's disease. *Disability and Rehabilitation, 31,* 1925-1936.

Remers, L., Widmeyer, W. N., Williams, J. M., and Meyers, L. (1995). Possible mediators and moderators of the class size-member adherence relationship in exercise. *Journal of Applied Sport Psychology, 7*, 38-49.

Resnick, B., Orwig, D., Magaziner, J., and Wynne, C. (2002). The effect of social support on exercise behavior in older adults. *Clinical Nursing Research, 11*, 52-70.

Rimmer, J. H., Riley, B., Wang, E., Rauworth, A., and Jurkowski, J. (2004). Physical activity participation among persons with disabilities. *American Journal of Preventive Medicine, 26*, 419-425.

Robbins, L B., Stommel, M., and Hamel, L. M. (2008). Social support for physical activity of middle school students. *Public Health Nursing, 25*, 451-460.

Rovniak, L. S., Anderson, E. S., Winett, R. A., and Stephens, R. S. (2002). Social cognitive determinants of physical activity in young adults: A prospective structural equation analysis. *Annals of Behavioral Medicine, 24*, 149-156.

Sabiston, C. M., McDonough, M. H., and Crocker, P. R. E. (2007). Psychosocial experiences of breast cancer survivors involved in a dragon boat program: Exploring links to positive psychological growth. *Journal of Sport and Exercise Psychology, 29*, 419-438.

Sallis, J. F., Prochaska, J. J., and Taylor, W. C. (2000). A review of correlates of physical activity of children and adolescents. *Medicine and Science in Sports and Exercise, 32*, 963-975.

Schutzer, K. A., and Graves, B. S. (2004). Barriers and motivation to exercise in older adults. *Preventive Medicine, 39*, 1056-1061.

Sinden, A. R., Martin Ginis, K. A., and Angove, J. (2003). Older women's reactions to revealing and nonrevealing exercise attire. *Journal of Aging and Physical Activity, 11*, 445-458.

Spink, K. S., and Carron, A. V. (1992). Group cohesion and adherence in exercise classes. *Journal of Sport and Exercise Psychology, 14*, 78-86.

Spink, K. S., and Carron, A. V. (1993). The effects of team building on the adherence patterns of female exercise participants. *Journal of Sport and Exercise Psychology, 15*, 39-49.

Spink, K. S., and Carron, A. V. (1994). Group cohesion effects in exercise classes. *Small Group Research, 25*, 26-42.

Szumilewicz, A. (2011). Multiple influences affecting the women's choice of a fitness club. *Baltic Journal of Health and Physical Activity, 3*, 55-64.

Taylor, W. C., Baranowski, T., and Sallis, J. F. (1994). Family determinants of childhood physical activity: A social-cognitive model. In R. K. Dishman (Ed.), *Advances in exercise adherence* (pp. 319-342). Champaign, IL: Human Kinetics.

Thoits, P. A. (2011). Mechanisms linking social ties and support to physical and mental health. *Journal of Health and Social Behavior, 52*, 145-161.

Trost, S. G., Owen, N., Bauman, A. E., Sallis, J. F., and Brown, W. (2002). Correlates of adults' participation in physical activity: Review and update. *Medicine and Science in Sports and Exercise, 34*, 1996-2001.

Turner, E. E., Rejeski, W. J., and Brawley, L. R. (1997). Psychological benefits of physical activity are influenced by the social environment. *Journal of Sport and Exercise Psychology, 19*, 119-130.

Unruh, A. M., and Elvin, N. (2004). In the eye of the dragon: Women's experience of breast cancer and the occupation of dragon boat racing. *Canadian Journal of Occupational Therapy, 71*, 138-149.

Voorhees, C. C., Murray, D., Welk, G., Birnbaum, A., Ribisl, K. M., Johnson, C. C., Pfeiffer, K. A., Saksvig, B., and Jobe, J. B. (2005). The role of peer social network factors and physical activity in adolescent girls. *American Journal of Health Behavior, 29*, 183-190.

Watson, J. D., Martin Ginis, K. A., and Spink, K. S. (2006). Team building in an exercise class for the elderly. *Activities, Adaptation and Aging, 28*, 35-47.

Wilcox, S., King, A. C., Brassington, G. S., and Ahn, D. K. (1999). Physical activity preferences of middle-aged and older adults: A community analysis. *Journal of Aging and Physical Activity, 7*, 386-399.

Wilson, K. S., and Spink, K. S. (2006). Exploring older adults' social influences for physical activity. *Activities, Adaptation and Aging, 30*, 47-60.

Wolinsky, F. D., Stump, T. E., and Clark, D. O. (1995). Antecedents and consequences of physical activity and exercise among older adults. *The Gerontologist, 35*, 451.

In: Positive Human Functioning ... Volume 2 ISBN: 978-1-62948-973-5
Editors: A. R. Gomes, R. Resende and A. Albuquerque © 2014 Nova Science Publishers, Inc.

Chapter 8

EXERCISE AND ITS RELATIONSHIP TO PSYCHOLOGICAL HEALTH AND WELL-BEING

Ali A. Weinstein[1], Susan E. Lydick[2] and Sukanya Biswabharati[3]
[1] Center for the Study of Chronic Illness and Disability,
College of Health and Human Services, George Mason University, Virginia, US
[2] Department of Rehabilitation Science,
College of Health and Human Services, George Mason University, Virginia, US
[3] Department of Psychology and Biology, Faculty of Science,
McMaster University, Ontario, Canada

ABSTRACT

This chapter will focus on the psychological health benefits of exercise and physical activity. Throughout this chapter, the terms exercise and physical activity will be used interchangeably. The majority of previous literature has focused on the relationship between exercise and its effect on mood disorders and anxiety. These relationships will be reviewed. However, exercise and physical activity have stress management, well-being, and flow experience implications to the general population, as well. The proper "dosing" of exercise can be an important key to maximizing the mental health benefits of exercise and therefore the literature on type, duration, intensity and frequency of exercise will also be discussed. At the conclusion of this chapter potential mechanisms that may explain the relationship between exercise and psychological health are discussed within two broad and overlapping categories: psychological and physiological mechanisms.

INTRODUCTION

Physical activity is recommended to the general population by many medical entities, including the Centers for Disease Control in the United States and the American College of Sports Medicine because it is considered an important tool for the improvement of public health (Garber et al., 2011; Pate et al., 1995). Based on the evidence, physical activity promotes health and is useful for the prevention of and treatment of a variety of diseases, including heart disease (Leon, Connett, Jacobs, and Rauramaa, 1987; Morris, Clayton, Everitt, Semmence, and Burgess, 1990; Paffenbarger, Hyde, Wing, and Hsieh, 1986), hypertension (Blair, Goodyear, Gibbons, and Cooper, 1984; Paffenbarger, Wing, Hyde, and Jung, 1983), non-insulin dependent diabetes (Helmrich, Ragland, Leung, and Paffenbarger, 1991; Manson et al., 1991, 1992), and osteoporosis (Carter et al., 2002; Marcus et al., 1992; Prior, Barr, Chow, and Faulkner, 1996).

In addition, there is a substantial body of evidence that shows a positive relationship between physical activity and mental health and illness (Biddle and Mutrie, 2001; Callaghan, 2004; Fontaine, 2000). The focus of this chapter will be on these psychological health benefits of exercise. When psychological health benefits are mentioned, it is important to put into perspective that individual's with a diagnosis of mental illness are not the only beneficiaries of the positive mental health benefits of exercise and physical activity. Mental illnesses lie on a continuum of level of symptomatology and even a mild amount of symptoms can have serious impact on individual happiness (Horwath, Johnson, Klerman, and Weissman, 1994). Exercise can not only decrease negative affect, but also potentially increase positive affect. Individuals with sub-clinical levels of symptoms would not usually be treated with pharmacotherapy. It may be increasingly important for individuals with subclinical symptomatology (within the normal range of mood variability) to use exercise and physical activity as "self-medication" to normalize mood state.

Relationship of Exercise to Mental Health Constructs

Depressive Symptoms

Depression is a major concern for many individuals as it can significantly impact physical and mental well-being as well as interpersonal and occupational functioning. Mental ailments such as mood disorders and clinical depression have been identified as some of the leading contributors to the global disease burden (Murray and Lopez, 1997) and a major cause of disability (Parikh, Lam, and CANMAT Depression Work Group, 2001). Cross-sectional studies have consistently demonstrated an association between habitual exercise level and low depressive symptoms levels (Ruuskanen and Ruoppila, 1995). Aerobic exercise 3 to 5 days a week at the recommended public health dose (17.5Kcal/Kg/week) was shown to be an effective therapy for mild to moderate major depressive disorder (MDD) in adults aged 20 to 45. Moreover, the response and remission rate was found to be comparable to other available depression treatments, such as medication or cognitive behavioral therapy (Dunn, Trivedi, Kampert, Clark, and Chambliss, 2005). Blumenthal et al. (1999) found that 16 weeks of group exercise training in patients with Major Depressive Disorder was as effective as anti-depressant medication (sertraline) (Blumenthal et al., 1999). Most remarkable is that at the 10-month follow-up point, the relapse rate was significantly lower in the exercise group compared to the other treatment arms (Babyak et al., 2000). Furthermore, this inverse relationship between physical activity and depression has been shown to be independent of possible confounding factors such as gender and socioeconomic status (Penedo and Dahn, 2005). In general, physical activity has benefited individuals with mood disorders, including depression (Martinsen, 1990).

Anxiety

Compared to the wide range of research on the positive effects of exercise in depression, anxiety disorders have been less frequently studied (Ströhle, 2009). However, a growing body of literature indicates that aerobic exercise is an effective and cost-efficient treatment for a variety of anxiety disorders including generalized anxiety and panic disorder (Salmon, 2001).

The use of exercise as a means to lower anxiety levels has shown to be advantageous for clinical as well as non-clinical participants (Long and Stavel, 1995; Rothman, 2010). Also, sub-clinical adults with a high state-anxiety show a reduction in anxiety after chronic and acute levels of exercise (Long and Stavel, 1995). Moreover, exercise is especially effective for adults who feel more anxious due to higher levels of stressful situations (Salmon, 2001).

Exercise also leads to a reduction in levels of anxiety in patients with other mental disorders (Long and Stavel, 1995). For example, obsessive compulsive disorder (OCD) is associated with symptoms of anxiety and depression and exercise has shown to reduce both symptoms of anxiety and depression in individuals with OCD (Lancer, Motta, and Lancer, 2007). Patients with anxiety disorders and dysphoric moods experience lower amounts of anxiety after a bout of physical exercise that is comparable to reductions in anxiety with the use of pharmacotherapy and cognitive therapy (Otto and Smits, 2011). The results for the reductions in anxiety with exercise may be partially explained through "exposure" to feared physiological sensations (i.e., high heart rate, rapid breathing). Therefore, in the context of anxiety, exercise may be acting as a desensitization technique for individuals with panic attacks or generalized anxiety that tend to misinterpret and catastrophize physiological sensations (Broman-Fulks, Berman, Rabian, and Webster, 2004).

Stress

Surprisingly, little is known about the stress-regulatory role of physical exercise (Klaperski, von Dawans, Heinrichs, and Fuchs, 2013). In the literature, one of the most discussed assumptions is that exercise might influence the stress system via its stress-buffering effects (a hypothesis). Exercise is thought to act as a moderator of the stress-health relationship by reducing the detrimental effects of chronic stress on both physical and mental health (Gerber, Kellmann, Hartmann, and Pühse, 2010; Tsatsoulis and Fountoulakis, 2006). Another possibility is that regular exercise may produce a more beneficial cardiovascular and endocrine stress response that in turn improves both mental and physical health outcome (Hamer, Taylor, and Steptoe, 2006; Sothmann et al., 1996).

Stress, although an issue in itself, causes numerous other psychological and physical issues that can negatively impact humans. These can include turning to unhealthy habits such as drinking, smoking and substance abuse, as well as being prone to multiple psychological diseases (Tavolacci et al., 2013). Low-fitness individuals had poorer physical health due to life-stressors compared to high-fitness individuals who had little impact on their physical health due to life-stressors (Roth and Holmes, 1987). Moreover, a study of a group of people who were HIV positive found that the ones who trained physically showed lower amounts of emotional distress as well as reduced decline of natural killer cells of the immune system compared to the non-training group (LaPerriere et al., 1990). In summary, a recent review found consistent evidence for exercise-based stress reduction and endorses exercise as a stress-management strategy (Gerber and Pühse, 2009).

Flow

Flow is a state of consciousness in which an individual has absolute concentration and is completely absorbed in an activity being performed. While in "flow", individuals experience an exhilarating feeling of transcendence; emotional problems seem to disappear, people feel strong and alert, at the peak of their abilities (Csikszentmihalyi, 1991).

Research has further indicated that for people to experience flow, there needs to be an optimal combination of personal skills and external challenges (Csikszentmihalyi, 1975). When an individual perceives the challenge and their available skills as both high and in balance, then a state of flow (highly intrinsically motivating) can be experienced (Csikszentmihalyi and Csikszentmihalyi, 1992). The majority of the research has focused on the experiences of athletes in connection with peak performance, but experiencing flow does not necessarily have to go along with athletic peak performances (Jackson and Csikszentmihalyi, 1999). Routine exercise or physical activity could be activities that induce flow. In one investigation, it was demonstrated that flow was induced by a running intervention for individuals with depression (Reinhardt et al., 2008). It has also been demonstrated that sedentary individuals involved in a physical activity intervention can also experience flow experiences (Elbe, Strahler, Krustrup, Wikman, and Stelter, 2010). Eliciting flow during exercise is intrinsically motivating for participants and is hypothesized to positively influence mental health and long-term adherence to physical activity (Schüler and Brunner, 2009).

Psychological Well-Being

Exercise not only assists in reducing depression in clinical as well as sub-clinical populations but also leads to a general improvement in mental functioning and provides a sense of psychological well-being (Biddle and Fox, 2000). Self-esteem is often seen to be the single most important component of psychological well-being. Self-esteem refers to the value placed on aspects of the self. Research has demonstrated an increase in self-esteem from participation in physical activity as well as increases in fitness (Sonstroem, 1984). A review identified 36 randomized controlled trials investigating the relationship between self-esteem and exercise. It was found that 76% of these trials resulted in positive changes in physical self-perceptions or general self-esteem (Fox, 2000). Therefore, exercise can be used to promote positive increases in self-esteem. Moreover, children and adolescents also experience improved significant changes in their perception of self following participation in exercise programs (Ekeland, Heian, Hagen, Abbott, and Nordheim, 2004). Another benefit of exercise is increased levels of self-reported happiness (Stubbe, de Moor, Boomsma, and de Geus, 2007).

Life satisfaction refers to a person's judgment of the quality o f their accomplishments and their current life circumstances (Diener, 1984). Several studies have examined the relationship between physical activity and life satisfaction (McAuley, Elavsky, Jerome,

Konopack, and Marquez, 2005). There is a consistent, albeit small relationship between increased life satisfaction and engagement in exercise (Diener, 2012). This small relationship is consistent with the view that life satisfaction is complex web of causality. It would be too implausible for a large increase in life satisfaction to occur when only one area of life (physical activity) is modified (Emmons, 1986). Overall, there are data that support the idea that physical activity is related to selected components of psychological well-being (self-esteem, happiness, and life satisfaction).

Quality of Life

Most of the literature on the relationship between exercise and quality of life has been performed in patient populations (i.e., heart disease, major depressive disorder, cancer, stroke) (Mitchell and Barlow, 2011). However, in one recent study of a general population in Sweden, it was demonstrated that an improved quality of life was found in response to an exercise intervention (Eriksson et al., 2010). In a large randomized controlled trial examining the effects of exercise on quality of life, a dose-response relationship was found (Martin, Church, Thompson, Earnest, and Blair, 2009). Therefore, a relationship existed between the amount of exercise performed and improvements in quality of life. These findings suggest that increasing physical activity is an effective tool for improving quality of life even in individuals without significant morbidities.

Cognitive Functioning

Cognitive functioning is an important component of psychological health and well-being and there have been many investigations looking at the relationship between cognitive functioning and exercise. A meta-analysis of 18 studies examining the effects of exercise on cognitive functioning in older adults found that exercise produced a moderate improvement in cognitive functioning (i.e., memory, perceptual organization) (Van Sickle, Hersen, Simco, Melton, and Hasselt, 1996). Another meta-analysis studying the effects of exercise on cognitive functioning analyzed results from 134 studies. The effect sizes of the most well-designed studies revealed a small, but significant increase in cognitive functioning, even within a younger aged population (Etnier et al., 1997). There is consistent evidence that exercise is beneficial to cognitive functioning (Callaghan, 2004).

Characteristics of Exercise to Enhance Psychological Benefits

This section will focus on the exercise structures that can influence the psychological benefits achieved via exercise. The four main components of exercise are intensity, duration, frequency and modality (or type of exercise). These factors can have huge impacts on the psychological outcomes of exercise.

Intensity

Moderate or low-intensity exercise has been demonstrated to be superior to high-intensity exercise for improving mood. Moreover, high-intensity exercise has been found to cause increased tension and fatigue despite prior fitness level (Ekkekakis, Parfitt, and Petruzzello, 2011). When exercise intensity requires a transition to anaerobic metabolism (high intensity), negative affect was generated (Hall, Ekkekakis, and Petruzzello, 2002). These negative feelings to seem to rebound after the exercise, however these transient periods of negative affect could reduce adherence to exercise programs. In fact, it appears that a curvilinear dose-response relationship between affect and intensity exists. Moderate training intensities resulted in immediate, large, and enduring affective benefits, while high and low intensity exercise did not show these same affective benefits (Arent, Landers, Matt, and Etnier, 2005). Additionally, individuals report a feeling of optimism after moderate-intensity training, especially in those who were relatively unhappy or depressed initially (Salmon, 2001).

Type of Exercise/Physical Activity (Modality)

Considering the options available for types of exercises (i.e., anaerobic vs. aerobic, Tai chi, yoga) it can be difficult to define the most beneficial alternative. Although aerobic exercises, have been the focus of much of the literature, anaerobic exercise regimens have been found equally effective as mood enhancer (Scully, Kremer, Meade, Graham, and Dudgeon, 1998). Nevertheless, in non-habitual exercises, anaerobic exercises have sometimes been shown to lead to a negative mood state. This might be because non-exercisers find strenuous exercises unpleasant. Due to these inconsistencies in the literature in respect to anaerobic exercises, aerobic exercises are mostly recommended (Salmon, 2001).

It is important to remember that common sense would suggest that people are happiest when they are doing an activity they like. Research has supported this notion. Individuals given a choice of type of exercise exhibit higher levels of positive affect after the exercise bout in comparison to individuals without a choice, even when the exercise intensity levels are held constant (Daley and Maynard, 2003).

Duration

Studies have shown that exercisers can obtain mood benefits form as little as 10 minutes of aerobic activity (Hansen, Stevens, and Coast, 2001). However, to reiterate from the discussion above, a person's self-selection of duration is an important component of the mood enhancement following exercise (Szabo, 2003). The positive effects of exercise are related to the duration of the training which includes both the entire period of training as well as the individual length of each session (Craft and Landers, 1998). For example, individuals exercising for 12 weeks showed largest reductions in depression compared to individuals training for 8 weeks (Craft and Landers, 1998). Therefore, longer exercise programs are associated with larger decreases in depressive symptoms. Also, individuals who continued the exercise regimen, aerobic or anaerobic, even after termination of a year program had a lower depression score compared to sedentary individuals (Scully et al., 1998).

Frequency

There are even fewer studies that have examined the effects of different exercise frequencies on psychological functioning McAuley (1991) found that a higher frequency of regular physical activity yielded higher levels of positive affect (McAuley, 1991). In addition, a higher frequency of exercise is associated with less depressive symptomatology (Conroy, Smith, and Felthous, 1982; Hassmén, Koivula, and Uutela, 2000). These results, taken as a whole, suggest that the more frequent the bouts of exercise, the larger the improvement in psychological health.

Psychological Mechanisms for Exercise-Induced Psychological Health

Self-Esteem and Self-Efficacy

Exercise induced increases in self-esteem and self-efficacy are widely acclaimed psychosocial processes and outcomes believed to be key to mechanisms involved in the antidepressant and mood-enhancing effects of exercise. Bandura (2001) posited that the best source of self-efficacy information comes from meaningful mastery experiences and researchers hypothesize that exercise can be such a meaningful mastery experience (Bandura, 2001). Ryan (2008, 2010) provides strong empirical evidence for this hypothesis by utilizing structural equation modeling (SEM) as a means to assess and expand upon the Exercise and Self Esteem Model (Sonstroem, 1984). Ryan reports that among the undergraduate college students (ages 18-25) he studied, results of SEM demonstrated that aerobic activity was associated with perceived endurance, which was in turn positively associated with physical esteem, which was in turn positively associated with global esteem. The salience of physical appearance and body image is likely increased within the United States culture where this study was conducted. Therefore, it is logical that the physical aspects of esteem account for significant variance in global esteem and thus personal sense of well-being. Although global esteem was negatively associated with depressive symptoms for males, it was not for females. Therefore, as Ryan hypothesized esteem is only part of the mechanism involved in the antidepressant process of exercise.

Efficacy surrounding exercise or belief that one can do exercise is also important. Ryan's SEM demonstrated that reported physical activity level was positively associated with the task efficacy subscale which includes items to assess responder confidence in their ability to complete an aerobic exercise session. Physical activity was also positively associated with the Scheduling Efficacy subscale conceptualized as goal setting and planning behaviors that promote exercise adherence. Perhaps the most interesting of Ryan's findings was that scheduling efficacy was negatively associated with depressive symptoms where task efficacy was not negatively associated with depressive symptoms. These data are counter to Bodin and Martinsen's hypothesis that increases in task efficacy is the mechanism by which exercise has antidepressant effects (Bodin and Martinsen, 2004) but provide support for Craft and Lander's hypothesis that increases in self-regulatory efficacy (akin to scheduling efficacy) is the primary mechanism that accounts for the antidepressant effects of exercise (Craft and Landers, 1998).

Thus when a person is successful in developing a plan of action for a particular exercise goal or outcome, is able to self-monitor exercise behaviors, use social support to maintain positive exercise behaviors, carry out the plan of action and achieve the intended physical activity or fitness outcome despite challenges and obstacles, the person is likely to feel exercise self-efficacy in particular and coping self-efficacy more generally. Thus the antidepressant effects of PA may result via increased feelings of scheduling *or* self-regulatory self-efficacy.

Self-Image Hypothesis

A related hypothesis to the self-esteem/self-efficacy hypothesis is the self-image hypothesis. This hypothesis suggests that the positive association between exercise and mental health is due to the favorable effects of exercise on body weight and body structure, resulting in more positive feedback from peer groups, which in turn improves an individual's self-image (Kirkcaldy, Shephard, and Siefen, 2002). This improvement in self-image results in mood enhancement (Monshouwer, Have, Poppel, Kemper, and Vollebergh, 2012). Studies that specifically test this hypothesis are not prevalent, but there is literature demonstrating that physical activity is associated with a more positive body image (Hausenblas and Fallon, 2002) and those reporting that a more positive body image is associated with better mental health (Stice, Hayward, Cameron, Killen, and Taylor, 2000; ter Bogt et al., 2006).

Distraction

Researchers hypothesize that the distraction from worries, anxiety, and depressing thoughts provided by exercise may be another psychological mechanism for exercise-induced psychological health (Bahrke and Morgan, 1978). This hypothesis seems quite consistent with the concept of flow and the intense cognitive and perceptual attention concentration required for a flow experience. Despite continuing references in the literature to the distraction hypothesis there does not seem to be strong empirical support for the hypothesis. Craft concluded in a quasi-experimental study in which clinically depressed women self-selected into either the control or 9 week exercise intervention that although exercisers ruminated less than non-exercisers, distraction could not account for antidepressant effects of exercise (Craft, 2005). However, in an investigation comparing meditation (quiet, distracting activity) and exercise (arousing, distracting activity), both activities induced mood enhancement via distracting processes (Bahrke and Morgan, 1978). Therefore, it is suggested that distraction may account for some of the antidepressant effects of exercise (Paluska and Schwenk, 2000). It may also be that a flow experience is necessary for the individual to truly feel "distracted." Additional research on this potential connection is needed.

Social Interaction

The social interaction hypothesis postulates that the social relationships and mutual support which exercisers provide each other accounts for a substantial portion of the effects of exercise on mental health (Greist et al., 1979). In contrast, other studies have failed to support this hypothesis and found mood enhancement without the social interaction component (Glenister, 1996). A focused review of this potential mechanism failed to support this social interaction hypothesis as the *primary* mediator of the mood-enhancing properties of exercise. But, it may have some important predictive power for adherence to an exercise program, especially in the early stages of adaption (North, McCullagh, and Tran, 1990).

PHYSIOLOGICAL MECHANISMS FOR EXERCISE-INDUCED PSYCHOLOGICAL HEALTH

Cerebral Blood Flow

Increases in cerebral blood flow with aerobic exercise has been widely studied (Ide and Secher, 2000). Enhanced blood flow to brain regions involved in the regulation of emotion could mediate changes in mood with exercise. In addition, researchers hypothesize that maintenance and/or restoration of cognitive functioning demonstrated among physically active as compared to sedentary adults, appears likely to be due at least in part to increased cerebral blood flow (Brown et al., 2010; Endo et al., 2013). This increased blood flow is thought to allow increased metabolic support to neurons that in turn allows the preservation of existing neurons, or increased development of new neurons. This line of research suggests that cognitive vitality, as well as mood enhancement, may be at least in part due to the increased blood flow proposed mechanism. However, there is currently little evidence to support the role of cerebral blood flow in mediating these effects in humans as most of the research has been conducted in animal models (O'Neal, Dunn, and Martinsen, 2000).

Neurogenesis

Exercise can increase the synthesis of new neurons in adult brains. Specifically, the hippocampal area of the brain seems to be highly involved in human emotion and psychological functioning (Ernst, Olson, Pinel, Lam, and Christie, 2006). Erickson et al. provide further support for the increased neurogenesis as a result of aerobic exercise in their study that found increased hippocampal volume as measured by magnetic resonance imaging in a moderate aerobic exercise group and hippocampal volume loss in the non-aerobic exercise group over a 6 month three day per week intervention (Erickson et al., 2011). There are several candidate molecules that could play a role in this hypothesized exercise-induced neurogenesis: β-endorphins, vascular endothelial growth factor (VEGF), brain-derived neurotrophic factor (BDNF), and serotonin (5-HT).

β-endorphins

An increase in β-endorphins after exercise was first reported over 20 years ago, when researchers believed that β-endorphins explained addictions to exercise of the "runner's high" (Colt, Wardlaw, and Frantz, 1981; Farrell, Gates, Maksud, and Morgan, 1982; Gambert et al., 1981). Although, enthusiasm for that interpretation has waned considerably, there is growing evidence that β-endorphins may play a role in neurogenesis. Recent results have implicated β-endorphins in the genesis (or perhaps survival) of new neurons in the hippocampus (Overstreet et al., 2004).

Vascular Endothelial Growth Factor

VEGF is another molecule that may link exercise and adult neurogenesis (Fabel et al., 2003). VEGF is increased when individuals exercise, and the simple infusion of this molecule (in the absence of exercise) increases neurogenesis in adult rats (Jin et al., 2002; Schobersberger et al., 2000). Specifically, VEGF seems to induce neurogenesis specifically in the hippocampal regions, implicating it in the mood enhancing qualities of exercise (Ernst et al., 2006).

Brain-Derived Neurotrophic Factor

Exercise leads to increased BDNF (Berchtold, Kesslak, Pike, Adlard, and Cotman, 2001; Neeper, Gómez-Pinilla, Choi, and Cotman, 1996; Russo-Neustadt, Beard, and Cotman, 1999). BDNF plays a critical role by promoting neuronal survival and regeneration of cells in the hippocampal region. Therefore, exercise is an effective strategy for increasing BDNF. In turn, the increased BDNK may enhance the survival of new cells in the hippocampal region (Cotman and Berchtold, 2002).

Serotonin

Exercise elevates levels of 5-HT precursors within the brain stem that sends projections to the hippocampus and therefore influences hippocampal activity (Chaouloff, Laude, and Elghozi, 1989). Although the precursors to 5-HT (i.e., tryptophan) are elevated in response to exercise, there is a lack of data that explicitly demonstrates an increase in 5-HT. However, theoretically, an increased expression of tryptophan might enhance 5-HT production and augment neurogenesis (Ernst et al., 2006).

Thermogenesis

Increased core body temperature as a result of exercise is another hypothesis for a mechanism involved in the mood enhancement and relaxation benefits of exercise. However, results have been inconsistent (Fox, 1999). This thermogenic model suggests that the body temperature elevations reduce tonic muscle activity, which in turn reduces somatic anxiety (deVries, Wiswell, Bulbulian, and Moritani, 1981; Petruzzello, Landers, and Salazar, 1993). This reduction in somatic anxiety is hypothesized to cause the mood improvements after exercise. During physical activity, the core body temperature is elevated. deVries et al. (1993) hypothesizes that these increases in temperature affect specific brain regions, such as the brain stem, which leads to a reduction in muscular tension and increasing an overall feeling of relaxation. At the current state of the literature, it seems reasonable that this hypothesis may explain part of the mood enhancing qualities of exercise, but more research is needed to specifically investigate the thermogenic hypothesis (Martinsen, 1990).

Analgesia

Physical exercise has been shown to suppress pain and induce sedation but the underlying mechanisms are still being investigated. Activation of the endorphin system was previously considered a major hypothesis for the mechanism explaining the analgesic qualities of exercise. A current hypothesis is that exercise activates the endocannabinoid system and thus induces analgesia and sedation and anxiolysis (Sparling, Giuffrida, Piomelli, Rosskopf, and Dietrich, 2003). Support for this hypothesis comes from the increased anandamide levels in blood samples taken (viewed as a marker of endocannabinoid system activation) from runners and cyclists but not sedentary controls following a 1-hour moderate exercise protocol (Sparling et al., 2003). This exercise-induced suppression of pain would then lead to mood-enhancement (Trivedi, 2004).

Attenuation of Stress Responsivity

As discussed earlier, exercise has been associated with reduced reactivity to stress. Rimmele, Seler, Marti, Wirtz, Ehlert, and Heinrsichs (2009) report as others have that that physically fit adults show attenuated hypothalamopituitary adrenal responses to both physical and mental stressors as measured by cortisol, heart rate, and state anxiety (Rimmele et al., 2009). This attenuation is seen as a quieting of the stress response system.

Cortisol is implicated as the mechanism for the negative affect experienced during physical or psychosocial stress situations and considered a marker of perceived uncontrollability, distress and helplessness (Webb et al., 2013). If exercise training results in attenuated HPA axis activation and cortisol release then individuals may experience less physiological responsiveness and mood detriment to stressful situations. In addition, this may be the common mastery experience mechanism (discussed within the psychological mechanisms section above) whereby exercise provides the opportunity to experience self-efficacy or control over physiological reactivity to stressors. There is some support for this hypothesis as self-efficacy has been found to be associated with lower anxiety and attenuated stress reactivity (Butki, Rudolph, and Jacobsen, 2001).

SUMMARY OF POTENTIAL MECHANISMS

Much more research is needed to fully understand the psychological and physiological mechanisms that may explain the psychological benefits of engaging in regular exercise. Future studies would benefit from integrative psychobiological models (incorporating both psychological and physiological measures/constructs) tested within the same prospective studies with both healthy and clinical adult populations. Despite the need for further research there is a evidence that strongly suggests that engagement in aerobic exercise during adulthood promotes blood flow to the brain, has a role in supporting neurogenesis, and contributes feelings of mastery and efficacy when the exercise is challenging and personally meaningful.

KEY POINTS TO PROMOTE POSITIVE HUMAN FUNCTIONING

Although this chapter has highlighted many areas in the literature that are in need of clarification and further investigation, there are still clear conclusions that may be drawn. From this brief review, it is clear that there are psychological health advantages of exercise in addition to the well-established physiological health benefits. Certainly, for mental conditions such as depression and anxiety, exercise can serve in a therapeutic role. In addition, individuals without mental conditions can also have psychological benefits in response to exercise. There are key factors to remember that may help to enhance positive human functioning in response to exercise. These include:

1) Exercising at a moderate intensity level. The exercise should be challenging yet still within a confortable range for the individual to garner the most psychological benefit.
2) Choosing an activity that is continuous and rhythmic (i.e., running, walking, yoga, swimming) may help to bolster the psychological benefits. This chapter discussed distraction as one of the potential important mechanisms linking exercise to psychological benefit. Continuous and rhythmic activity may increase the distracting qualities of exercise.
3) The self-selection of the frequency, modality, intensity, and duration of the exercise is a key component of increasing positive human functioning. However, this self-selection must be made within the parameter that for an activity to be intrinsically motivating (and thereby increase positive human functioning), it needs to be "challenging" to the individual. A balancing act then occurs, the individuals must be challenged but still maintain a level that is within their individualized comfort zone for optimal mood improvements to occur.

CONCLUSION

The controversies surrounding the available data on the effects of exercise on psychological health and well-being have led to some confusion on the part of clinicians as to when and how to use exercise as part of a treatment regimen. However, as can be derived from this chapter, it is clear that exercise has a positive impact on psychological health and well-being. Not only in individuals with existent mental health illnesses, but also among individuals within the normal spectrum of mental health. Exercise can both decrease negative affect as well as increase positive affect. The areas in need of much more research include the details of the exercise prescription (duration, intensity, frequency, and modality) that will help to induce psychological health. We have broad stroke recommendations, moderate intensity, increased frequency, self-selection of modality, but we do not have specific recommendations that can be made to individuals. In addition, we do not have clear mechanisms that explain the link between exercise and psychological health. These mechanistic studies are important because if the agents of action are identified, then exercise regimens can be designed to specifically increase those agents. Physical activity and exercise can play an important role as a simple, inexpensive, and effective technique for increasing psychological health and well-being.

REFERENCES

Arent, S., Landers, D., Matt, K., and Etnier, J. (2005). Dose-response and mechanistic issues in the resistance training and affect relationship. *Journal of Sport and Exercise Psychology*, *27*, 92–110.

Babyak, M., Blumenthal, J. A., Herman, S., Khatri, P., Doraiswamy, M., Moore, K., Krishnan, K. R. (2000). Exercise treatment for major depression: Maintenance of therapeutic benefit at 10 months. *Psychosomatic Medicine*, *62*(5), 633–638.

Bahrke, M. S., and Morgan, W. P. (1978). Anxiety reduction following exercise and meditation. *Cognitive Therapy and Research*, *2*(4), 323–333. doi:10.1007/BF01172650

Bandura, A. (2001). Social cognitive theory: An agentic perspective. *Annual Review of Psychology*, *52*(1), 1–26. doi:10.1146/annurev.psych.52.1.1

Berchtold, N. C., Kesslak, J. P., Pike, C. J., Adlard, P. A., and Cotman, C. W. (2001). Estrogen and exercise interact to regulate brain-derived neurotrophic factor mRNA and protein expression in the hippocampus. *The European journal of neuroscience*, *14*(12), 1992–2002.

Biddle, S., Fox, K. R., and Boutcher. (2000). *Physical Activity and Psychological Well-Being*. London; New York: Routledge.

Biddle, S., and Mutrie, N. (2001). *Psychology of Physical Activity: Determinants, Well-being, and Interventions*. New York, NY: Psychology Press.

Blair, S. N., Goodyear, N. N., Gibbons, L. W., and Cooper, K. H. (1984). Physical fitness and incidence of hypertension in healthy normotensive men and women. *JAMA*, *252*(4), 487–490.

Blumenthal, J. A., Babyak, M. A., Moore, K. A., Craighead, W. E., Herman, S., Khatri, P., Krishnan, K. R. (1999). Effects of exercise training on older patients with major depression. *Archives of Internal Medicine*, *159*(19), 2349–2356.

Bodin, T., and Martinsen, E. W. (2004). Mood and self-efficacy during acute exercise in clinical depression. A randomized, controlled study. *Journal of Sport and Exercise Psychology*, *26*(4), 623–633.

Broman-Fulks, J. J., Berman, M. E., Rabian, B. A., and Webster, M. J. (2004). Effects of aerobic exercise on anxiety sensitivity. *Behaviour Research and Therapy*, *42*(2), 125–136. doi:10.1016/S0005-7967(03)00103-7

Brown, A. D., McMorris, C. A., Longman, R. S., Leigh, R., Hill, M. D., Friedenreich, C. M., and Poulin, M. J. (2010). Effects of cardiorespiratory fitness and cerebral blood flow on cognitive outcomes in older women. *Neurobiology of Aging*, *31*(12), 2047–2057. doi:10.1016/j.neurobiolaging.2008.11.002

Butki, B. D., Rudolph, D. L., and Jacobsen, H. (2001). Self-efficacy, state anxiety, and cortisol responses to treadmill running. *Perceptual and Motor Skills*, *92*(3 Pt 2), 1129–1138.

Callaghan, P. (2004). Exercise: A neglected intervention in mental health care? *Journal of psychiatric and mental health nursing*, *11*(4), 476–483. doi:10.1111/j.1365-2850.2004.00751.x

Carter, N. D., Khan, K. M., McKay, H. A., Petit, M. A., Waterman, C., Heinonen, A., …Flicker, L. (2002). Community-based exercise program reduces risk factors for falls in 65- to 75-year-old women with osteoporosis: Randomized controlled trial. *Canadian Medical Association Journal*, *167*(9), 997–1004.

Chaouloff, F., Laude, D., and Elghozi, J. L. (1989). Physical exercise: Evidence for differential consequences of tryptophan on 5-HT synthesis and metabolism in central serotonergic cell bodies and terminals. *Journal of Neural Transmission*, *78*(2), 121–130.

Colt, E. W., Wardlaw, S. L., and Frantz, A. G. (1981). The effect of running on plasma beta-endorphin. *Life Sciences*, *28*(14), 1637–1640.

Conroy, R. W., Smith, K., and Felthous, A. R. (1982). The value of exercise on a psychiatric hospital unit. *Hospital and Community Psychiatry*, *33*(8), 641–645.

Cotman, C. W., and Berchtold, N. C. (2002). Exercise: A behavioral intervention to enhance brain health and plasticity. *Trends in Neurosciences*, *25*(6), 295–301.

Craft, L. (2005). Exercise and clinical depression: Examining two psychological mechanisms. *Psychology of Sport and Exercise*, *6*(2), 151–171. doi:10.1016/j.psychsport.2003.11.003

Craft, L., and Landers, D. (1998). The effect of exercise on clinical depression and depression resulting from mental illness: A meta-analysis. *Journal of Sport and Exercise Psychology*, 339–357.

Csikszentmihalyi, M. (1975). *Beyond Boredom and Anxiety: Experiencing Flow in Work and Play*. San Francisco: Jossey-Bass Publishers.

Csikszentmihalyi, M. (1991). *Flow: The psychology of optimal experience*. New York, N.Y.: HarperPerennial.

Csikszentmihalyi, M., and Csikszentmihalyi, I. S. (1992). *Optimal Experience: Psychological Studies of Flow in Consciousness*. Cambridge; New York: Cambridge University Press.

Daley, A. J., and Maynard, I. W. (2003). Preferred exercise mode and affective responses in physically active adults. *Psychology of Sport and Exercise*, *4*(4), 347–356. doi:10.1016/S1469-0292(02)00018-3

deVries, H., Wiswell, R., Bulbulian, R., and Moritani, T. (1981). Tranquilizer effect of exercise: Acute effects of moderate aerobic exercise on spinal reflex activation level. *American Journal of Physical Medicine*, *60*(2), 57–66.

Diener, E. (1984). Subjective well-being. *Psychological Bulletin*, *95*(3), 542–575.

Diener, E. (2012). New findings and future directions for subjective well-being research. *The American Psychologist*, *67*(8), 590–597. doi:10.1037/a0029541

Dunn, A. L., Trivedi, M. H., Kampert, J. B., Clark, C. G., and Chambliss, H. O. (2005). Exercise treatment for depression: Efficacy and dose response. *American Journal of Preventive Medicine*, *28*(1), 1–8. doi:10.1016/j.amepre.2004.09.003

Ekeland, E., Heian, F., Hagen, K. B., Abbott, J., and Nordheim, L. (2004). Exercise to improve self-esteem in children and young people. *The Cochrane Database of Systematic Reviews*, (1), CD003683. doi:10.1002/14651858.CD003683.pub2

Ekkekakis, P., Parfitt, G., and Petruzzello, S. J. (2011). The pleasure and displeasure people feel when they exercise at different intensities: Decennial update and progress towards a tripartite rationale for exercise intensity prescription. *Sports Medicine*, *41*(8), 641–671. doi:10.2165/11590680-000000000-00000

Elbe, A., Strahler, K., Krustrup, P., Wikman, J., and Stelter, R. (2010). Experiencing flow in different types of physical activity intervention programs: Three randomized studies. *Scandinavian Journal of Medicine and Science in Sports*, *20 Suppl 1*, 111–117. doi:10.1111/j.1600-0838.2010.01112.x

Emmons, R. (1986). Personal strivings: An approach to personality and subjective well-being. *Journal of Personality and Social Psychology*, *51*(5), 1058–1068.

Endo, K., Matsukawa, K., Liang, N., Nakatsuka, C., Tsuchimochi, H., Okamura, H., and Hamaoka, T. (2013). Dynamic exercise improves cognitive function in association with increased prefrontal oxygenation. *The Journal of Physiological Sciences*, *63*(4), 287–298. doi:10.1007/s12576-013-0267-6

Erickson, K. I., Voss, M. W., Prakash, R. S., Basak, C., Szabo, A., Chaddock, L., Kramer, A. F. (2011). Exercise training increases size of hippocampus and improves memory. *Proceedings of the National Academy of Sciences*, *108*(7), 3017–3022. doi:10.1073/pnas.1015950108

Eriksson, M. K., Hagberg, L., Lindholm, L., Malmgren-Olsson, E.-B., Osterlind, J., and Eliasson, M. (2010). Quality of life and cost-effectiveness of a 3-year trial of lifestyle intervention in primary health care. *Archives of Internal Medicine*, *170*(16), 1470–1479. doi:10.1001/archinternmed.2010.301

Ernst, C., Olson, A. K., Pinel, J. P. J., Lam, R. W., and Christie, B. R. (2006). Antidepressant effects of exercise: Evidence for an adult-neurogenesis hypothesis? *Journal of Psychiatry and Neuroscience*, *31*(2), 84–92.

Etnier, J. L., Salazar, W., Landers, D. M., Petruzzello, S. J., Han, M., and Nowell, P. (1997). The influence of physical fitness and exercise upon cognitive functioning: A meta-analysis. *Journal of Sport and Exercise Psychology*, *19*(3), 249–277.

Fabel, K., Fabel, K., Tam, B., Kaufer, D., Baiker, A., Simmons, N., ... Palmer, T. D. (2003). VEGF is necessary for exercise-induced adult hippocampal neurogenesis. *The European Journal of Neuroscience*, *18*(10), 2803–2812.

Farrell, P. A., Gates, W. K., Maksud, M. G., and Morgan, W. P. (1982). Increases in plasma beta-endorphin/beta-lipotropin immunoreactivity after treadmill running in humans. *Journal of Applied Physiology: Respiratory, Environmental and Exercise Physiology*, *52*(5), 1245–1249.

Fontaine, K. R. (2000). Physical activity improves mental health. *The Physician and Sports Medicine*, *28*(10), 83–84. doi:10.3810/psm.2000.10.1256

Fox, K. R. (1999). The influence of physical activity on mental well-being. *Public Health Nutrition*, *2*(Supplement 3a), 411–418. doi:10.1017/S1368980099000567

Fox, K. R. (2000). Self-esteem, self-perceptions and exercise. *International Journal of Sport Psychology, 31*(2), 228–240.

Gambert, S. R., Garthwaite, T. L., Pontzer, C. H., Cook, E. E., Tristani, F. E., Duthie, E. H., McCarty, D. J. (1981). Running elevates plasma beta-endorphin immunoreactivity and ACTH in untrained human subjects. *Proceedings of the Society for Experimental Biology and Medicine, 168*(1), 1–4.

Garber, C. E., Blissmer, B., Deschenes, M. R., Franklin, B. A., Lamonte, M. J., Lee, I.-M., American College of Sports Medicine. (2011). American College of Sports Medicine position stand. Quantity and quality of exercise for developing and maintaining cardiorespiratory, musculoskeletal, and neuromotor fitness in apparently healthy adults: Guidance for prescribing exercise. *Medicine and Science in Sports and Exercise, 43*(7), 1334–1359. doi:10.1249/MSS.0b013e318213fefb

Gerber, M., Kellmann, M., Hartmann, T., and Pühse, U. (2010). Do exercise and fitness buffer against stress among Swiss police and emergency response service officers? *Psychology of Sport and Exercise, 11*(4), 286–294. doi:10.1016/j.psychsport.2010.02.004

Gerber, M., and Pühse, U. (2009). Do exercise and fitness protect against stress-induced health complaints? A review of the literature. *Scandinavian Journal of Public Health, 37*(8), 801–819. doi:10.1177/1403494809350522

Glenister, D. (1996). Exercise and mental health: A review. *Journal of the Royal Society of Health, 116*(1), 7–13.

Greist, J. H., Klein, M. H., Eischens, R. R., Faris, J., Gurman, A. S., and Morgan, W. P. (1979). Running as treatment for depression. *Comprehensive Psychiatry, 20*(1), 41–54.

Hall, E. E., Ekkekakis, P., and Petruzzello, S. J. (2002). The affective beneficence of vigorous exercise revisited. *British Journal of Health Psychology, 7*(Pt 1), 47–66. doi:10.1348/135910702169358

Hamer, M., Taylor, A., and Steptoe, A. (2006). The effect of acute aerobic exercise on stress related blood pressure responses: A systematic review and meta-analysis. *Biological Psychology, 71*(2), 183–190. doi:10.1016/j.biopsycho.2005.04.004

Hansen, C. J., Stevens, L. C., and Coast, J. R. (2001). Exercise duration and mood state: how much is enough to feel better? *Health Psychology, 20*(4), 267–275.

Hassmén, P., Koivula, N., and Uutela, A. (2000). Physical exercise and psychological well-being: A population study in Finland. *Preventive Medicine, 30*(1), 17–25. doi:10.1006/pmed.1999.0597

Hausenblas, H. A., and Fallon, E. A. (2002). Relationship among body image, exercise behavior, and exercise dependence symptoms. *The International Journal of Eating Disorders, 32*(2), 179–185. doi:10.1002/eat.10071

Helmrich, S. P., Ragland, D. R., Leung, R. W., and Paffenbarger, R. S., Jr. (1991). Physical activity and reduced occurrence of non-insulin-dependent diabetes mellitus. *The New England Journal of Medicine, 325*(3), 147–152. doi:10.1056/NEJM199107183250302

Horwath, E., Johnson, J., Klerman, G. L., and Weissman, M. M. (1994). What are the public health implications of subclinical depressive symptoms? *The Psychiatric Quarterly, 65*(4), 323–337.

Ide, K., and Secher, N. H. (2000). Cerebral blood flow and metabolism during exercise. *Progress in Neurobiology, 61*(4), 397–414. doi:10.1016/S0301-0082(99)00057-X

Jackson, S. A., and Csikszentmihalyi, M. (1999). *Flow in Sports*. Champaign, IL: Human Kinetics.

Jin, K., Zhu, Y., Sun, Y., Mao, X. O., Xie, L., and Greenberg, D. A. (2002). Vascular endothelial growth factor (VEGF) stimulates neurogenesis in vitro and in vivo. *Proceedings of the National Academy of Sciences of the United States of America*, *99*(18), 11946–11950. doi:10.1073/pnas.182296499

Kirkcaldy, B. D., Shephard, R. J., and Siefen, R. G. (2002). The relationship between physical activity and self-image and problem behaviour among adolescents. *Social Psychiatry and Psychiatric Epidemiology*, *37*(11), 544–550. doi:10.1007/s00127-002-0554-7

Klaperski, S., von Dawans, B., Heinrichs, M., and Fuchs, R. (2013). Does the level of physical exercise affect physiological and psychological responses to psychosocial stress in women? *Psychology of Sport and Exercise*, *14*(2), 266–274. doi:10.1016/j.psychsport.2012.11.003

Lancer, R., Motta, R., and Lancer, D. (2007). The effect of aerobic exercise on obsessive-compulsive disorder, anxiety, and depression: A preliminary investigation. *The Behavior Therapist*, *30*(3), 53, 57–62.

LaPerriere, A. R., Antoni, M. H., Schneiderman, N., Ironson, G., Klimas, N., Caralis, P., and Fletcher, M. A. (1990). Exercise intervention attenuates emotional distress and natural killer cell decrements following notification of positive serologic status for HIV-1. *Biofeedback and Self-regulation*, *15*(3), 229–242. doi:10.1007/BF01011107

Leon, A. S., Connett, J., Jacobs, D. R., Jr, and Rauramaa, R. (1987). Leisure-time physical activity levels and risk of coronary heart disease and death: The Multiple Risk Factor Intervention Trial. *JAMA*, *258*(17), 2388–2395.

Long, B. C., and Stavel, R. van. (1995). Effects of exercise training on anxiety: A meta-analysis. *Journal of Applied Sport Psychology*, *7*(2), 167–189. doi:10.1080/10413209508406963

Manson, J. E., Nathan, D. M., Krolewski, A. S., Stampfer, M. J., Willett, W. C., and Hennekens, C. H. (1992). A prospective study of exercise and incidence of diabetes among US male physicians. *JAMA*, *268*(1), 63–67.

Manson, J. E., Rimm, E. B., Stampfer, M. J., Colditz, G. A., Willett, W. C., Krolewski, A. S., Speizer, F. E. (1991). Physical activity and incidence of non-insulin-dependent diabetes mellitus in women. *Lancet*, *338*(8770), 774–778.

Marcus, R., Drinkwater, B., Dalsky, G., Dufek, J., Raab, D., Slemenda, C., and Snow-Harter, C. (1992). Osteoporosis and exercise in women. *Medicine and Science in Sports and Exercise*, *24*(6 Suppl), S301–307.

Martin, C. K., Church, T. S., Thompson, A. M., Earnest, C. P., and Blair, S. N. (2009). Exercise dose and quality of life: Results of a randomized controlled trial. *Archives of Internal Medicine*, *169*(3), 269–278. doi:10.1001/archinternmed.2008.545

Martinsen, D. E. W. (1990). Benefits of exercise for the treatment of depression. *Sports Medicine*, *9*(6), 380–389. doi:10.2165/00007256-199009060-00006

McAuley, E. (1991). Efficacy, attributional, and affective responses to exercise participation. *Journal of Sport and Exercise Psychology*, 382–393.

McAuley, E., Elavsky, S., Jerome, G. J., Konopack, J. F., and Marquez, D. X. (2005). Physical activity-related well-being in older adults: Social cognitive influences. *Psychology and Aging*, *20*(2), 295–302. doi:10.1037/0882-7974.20.2.295

Mitchell, T., and Barlow, C. E. (2011). Review of the role of exercise in improving quality of life in healthy individuals and in those with chronic diseases. *Current Sports Medicine Reports*, *10*(4), 211–216. doi:10.1249/JSR.0b013e318223cc9e

Monshouwer, K., Have, M. ten, Poppel, M. van, Kemper, H., and Vollebergh, W. (2012). Possible mechanisms explaining the association between physical activity and mental health: Findings From the 2001 Dutch Health Behaviour in School-Aged Children Survey. *Clinical Psychological Science*. doi:10.1177/2167702612450485

Morris, J. N., Clayton, D. G., Everitt, M. G., Semmence, A. M., and Burgess, E. H. (1990). Exercise in leisure time: Coronary attack and death rates. *British Heart Journal*, *63*(6), 325–334.

Murray, C. J., and Lopez, A. D. (1997). Global mortality, disability, and the contribution of risk factors: Global Burden of Disease Study. *Lancet*, *349*(9063), 1436–1442. doi:10.1016/S0140-6736(96)07495-8

Neeper, S. A., Gómez-Pinilla, F., Choi, J., and Cotman, C. W. (1996). Physical activity increases mRNA for brain-derived neurotrophic factor and nerve growth factor in rat brain. *Brain Research*, *726*(1-2), 49–56.

North, T. C., McCullagh, P., and Tran, Z. V. (1990). Effect of exercise on depression. *Exercise and Sport Sciences Reviews*, *18*, 379–415.

O'Neal, H. A., Dunn, A. L., and Martinsen, E. W. (2000). Depression and exercise. *International Journal of Sport Psychology*, *31*(2), 110–135.

Otto, M., and Smits, J. (2011). *Exercise for Mood and Anxiety: Proven Strategies for Overcoming Depression and Enhancing Well-Being*. New York, NY: Oxford University Press.

Overstreet, L. S., Hentges, S. T., Bumaschny, V. F., de Souza, F. S. J., Smart, J. L., Santangelo, A. M., Rubinstein, M. (2004). A transgenic marker for newly born granule cells in dentate gyrus. *The Journal of Neuroscience*, *24*(13), 3251–3259. doi:10.1523/JNEUROSCI.5173-03.2004

Paffenbarger, R. S., Jr, Hyde, R. T., Wing, A. L., and Hsieh, C. C. (1986). Physical activity, all-cause mortality, and longevity of college alumni. *The New England Journal of Medicine*, *314*(10), 605–613. doi:10.1056/NEJM198603063141003

Paffenbarger, R. S., Jr, Wing, A. L., Hyde, R. T., and Jung, D. L. (1983). Physical activity and incidence of hypertension in college alumni. *American Journal of Epidemiology*, *117*(3), 245–257.

Paluska, S. A., and Schwenk, T. L. (2000). Physical activity and mental health: Current concepts. *Sports Medicine*, *29*(3), 167–180.

Parikh, S. V., Lam, R. W., and CANMAT Depression Work Group. (2001). Clinical guidelines for the treatment of depressive disorders, I. Definitions, prevalence, and health burden. *Canadian Journal of Psychiatry*, *46 Suppl 1*, 13S–20S.

Pate, R. R., Pratt, M., Blair, S. N., Haskell, W. L., Macera, C. A., Bouchard, C., King, A. C. (1995). Physical activity and public health: A recommendation from the Centers for Disease Control and Prevention and the American College of Sports Medicine. *JAMA*, *273*(5), 402–407.

Penedo, F. J., and Dahn, J. R. (2005). Exercise and well-being: A review of mental and physical health benefits associated with physical activity. *Current Opinion in Psychiatry*, *18*(2), 189–193.

Petruzzello, S. J., Landers, D., and Salazar, W. (1993). Exercise and anxiety reduction: Examination of temperature as an explanation for affective change. *Journal of Sport and Exercise Psychology, 15*(1), 63–76.

Prior, J. C., Barr, S. I., Chow, R., and Faulkner, R. A. (1996). Prevention and management of osteoporosis: Consensus statements from the Scientific Advisory Board of the Osteoporosis Society of Canada. 5. Physical activity as therapy for osteoporosis. *Canadian Medical Association Journal, 155*(7), 940–944.

Reinhardt, C., Wiener, S., Heimbeck, A., Stoll, O., Lau, A., and Schliermann, R. (2008). Flow in der Sporttherapie der Depression – ein beanspruchungsorientierter Ansatz. *Bewegungstherapie und Gesundheitssport, 24*(04), 147–151. doi:10.1055/s-2008-1076899

Rimmele, U., Seiler, R., Marti, B., Wirtz, P. H., Ehlert, U., and Heinrichs, M. (2009). The level of physical activity affects adrenal and cardiovascular reactivity to psychosocial stress. *Psychoneuroendocrinology, 34*(2), 190–198. doi:10.1016/j.psyneuen.2008.08.023

Roth, D. L., and Holmes, D. S. (1987). Influence of aerobic exercise training and relaxation training on physical and psychologic health following stressful life events. *Psychosomatic Medicine, 49*(4), 355–365.

Rothman, M. T. (2010, December 31). *The Effect of Chronic Exercise on Trait Anxiety in College Students* (PhD). Emory University.

Russo-Neustadt, A., Beard, R. C., and Cotman, C. W. (1999). Exercise, antidepressant medications, and enhanced brain derived neurotrophic factor expression. *Neuropsychopharmacology, 21*(5), 679–682. doi:10.1016/S0893-133X(99)00059-7

Ruuskanen, J. M., and Ruoppila, I. (1995). Physical activity and psychological well-being among people aged 65 to 84 years. *Age and Ageing, 24*(4), 292–296.

Ryan, M. P. (2008). The antidepressant effects of physical activity: Mediating self-esteem and self-efficacy mechanisms. *Psychology and Health, 23*(3), 279–307. doi:10.1080/14768320601185502

Ryan, M. P. (2010). Psychocultural differences in physical activity-based antidepressant effects. *Mental Health and Physical Activity, 3*(1), 5–15. doi:10.1016/j.mhpa.2009.12.001

Salmon, P. (2001). Effects of physical exercise on anxiety, depression, and sensitivity to stress: A unifying theory. *Clinical Psychology Review, 21*(1), 33–61.

Schobersberger, W., Hobisch-Hagen, P., Fries, D., Wiedermann, F., Rieder-Scharinger, J., Villiger, B., ... Jelkmann, W. (2000). Increase in immune activation, vascular endothelial growth factor and erythropoietin after an ultramarathon run at moderate altitude. *Immunobiology, 201*(5), 611–620. doi:10.1016/S0171-2985(00)80078-9

Schüler, J., and Brunner, S. (2009). The rewarding effect of flow experience on performance in a marathon race. *Psychology of Sport and Exercise, 10*(1), 168–174. doi:10.1016/j.psychsport.2008.07.001

Scully, D., Kremer, J., Meade, M. M., Graham, R., and Dudgeon, K. (1998). Physical exercise and psychological well being: A critical review. *British Journal of Sports Medicine, 32*(2), 111–120.

Sonstroem, R. J. (1984). Exercise and self-esteem. *Exercise and Sport Sciences Reviews, 12*, 123–155.

Sothmann, M. S., Buckworth, J., Claytor, R. P., Cox, R. H., White-Welkley, J. E., and Dishman, R. K. (1996). Exercise training and the cross-stressor adaptation hypothesis. *Exercise and Sport Sciences Reviews, 24*, 267–287.

Sparling, P. B., Giuffrida, A., Piomelli, D., Rosskopf, L., and Dietrich, A. (2003). Exercise activates the endocannabinoid system. *Neuroreport*, *14*(17), 2209–2211. doi:10.1097/01.wnr.0000097048.56589.47

Stice, E., Hayward, C., Cameron, R. P., Killen, J. D., and Taylor, C. B. (2000). Body-image and eating disturbances predict onset of depression among female adolescents: A longitudinal study. *Journal of Abnormal Psychology*, *109*(3), 438–444.

Ströhle, A. (2009). Physical activity, exercise, depression and anxiety disorders. *Journal of Neural Transmission*, *116*(6), 777–784. doi:10.1007/s00702-008-0092-x

Stubbe, J. H., de Moor, M. H. M., Boomsma, D. I., and de Geus, E. J. C. (2007). The association between exercise participation and well-being: A co-twin study. *Preventive Medicine*, *44*(2), 148–152. doi:10.1016/j.ypmed.2006.09.002

Szabo, A. (2003). Acute psychological effects of exercise performed at self-selected workloads: Implications for theory and practice. *Journal of Sports Science and Medicine*, *2*, 77–87.

Tavolacci, M. P., Ladner, J., Grigioni, S., Richard, L., Villet, H., and Dechelotte, P. (2013). Prevalence and association of perceived stress, substance use and behavioral addictions: A cross-sectional study among university students in France, 2009-2011. *BMC Public Health*, *13*, 724. doi:10.1186/1471-2458-13-724

Ter Bogt, T. F. M., van Dorsselaer, S. A. F. M., Monshouwer, K., Verdurmen, J. E. E., Engels, R. C. M. E., and Vollebergh, W. A. M. (2006). Body mass index and body weight perception as risk factors for internalizing and externalizing problem behavior among adolescents. *The Journal of Adolescent Health*, *39*(1), 27–34. doi:10.1016/j.jadohealth.2005.09.007

Trivedi, M. H. (2004). The link between depression and physical symptoms. *Primary Care Companion to The Journal of Clinical Psychiatry*, *6*(suppl 1), 12–16.

Tsatsoulis, A., and Fountoulakis, S. (2006). The protective role of exercise on stress system dysregulation and comorbidities. *Annals of the New York Academy of Sciences*, *1083*, 196–213. doi:10.1196/annals.1367.020

Van Sickle, T. D., Hersen, M., Simco, E. R., Melton, M. A., and Hasselt, V. B. V. (1996). Effects of physical exercise on cognitive functioning in the elderly. *International Journal of Rehabilitation and Health*, *2*(2), 67–100. doi:10.1007/BF02213444

Webb, H. E., Rosalky, D. S., Tangsilsat, S. E., McLeod, K. A., Acevedo, E. O., and Wax, B. (2013). Aerobic fitness affects cortisol responses to concurrent challenges. *Medicine and Science in Sports and Exercise*, *45*(2), 379–386. doi:10.1249/MSS.0b013e318270b381

About the Editors

A. Rui Gomes

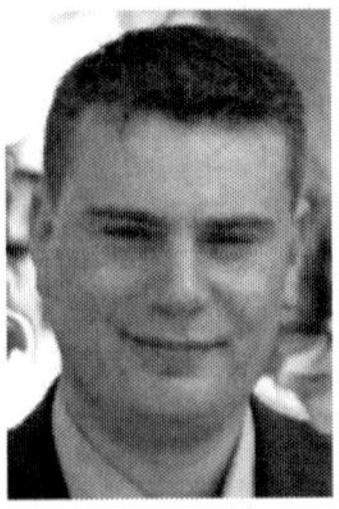

Department of Applied Psychology, School of Psychology, University of Minho, Portugal.
rgomes@psi.uminho.pt

Rui Gomes is an Assistant Professor in the School of Psychology at the University of Minho, Portugal. He performs research on two main areas: sport/exercise psychology (e.g., leadership, stress, psychological benefits of exercise, life skills training) and occupational stress (e.g., sources and consequences of stress in high-risk activities, impact of cognitive appraisal on human adaptation to stress). Currently, he leads the research group Adaptation, Performance and Human Development, which was created in 2007 (http://www.ardh-gi.com/). As a sport psychologist, he consults athletes and their families, coaches, and sport managers. Currently, he is the sport psychologist of the Bocce National Team.

Rui Resende

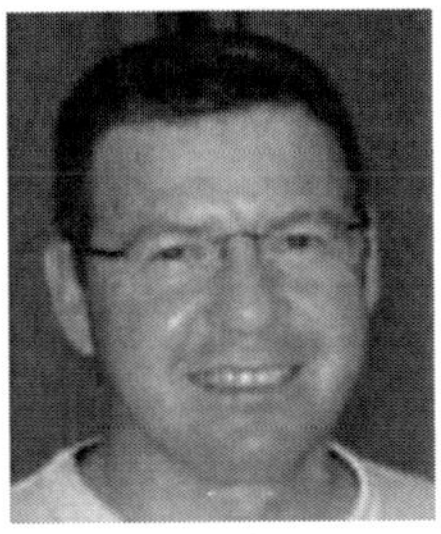

Maia Institute of Higher Education, Portugal
rresende@ismai.pt

Rui Resende is an Assistant Professor at the Maia Institute of Higher Education. He does research mainly in Coach Education. Presently, he is the Coordinator of the Master's program in Sports Performance and leads the investigative research line "Coaching and Education" in the research group Adaptation, Performance and Human Development. He was a volleyball athlete who won several national titles. He coached teams at the high competition level in Portugal and was also the junior national coach of the Portuguese team.

Alberto Albuquerque

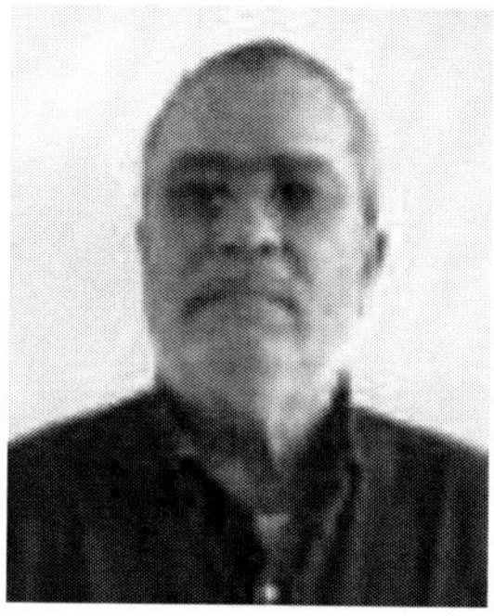

Maia Institute of Higher Education, Portugal
aalbuquerque@ismai.pt

Alberto Albuquerque is an Assistant Professor at the Maia Institute of Higher Education. His main area of research focuses on the factors involved in the education and training of physical education teachers. Currently, he is the coordinator of the Masters in Teaching Physical Education and the Supervised Teaching Practice.

He is a member of the Research Center in Sports Sciences, Health and Human Development, the Research Center in Sport and Physical Activity, and the research group Adaptation, Performance and Human Development.

He is co-founder and Chairman of the General Assembly of the Scientific Society of Sport Pedagogy. He is a member of the Portuguese Society of Physical Education and the Center for Continuous Education of the Maia Institute of Higher Education.

He collaborates as a reviewer with several international journals in the field of pedagogy.

About the Contributors

Preface

Kennon M. Sheldon

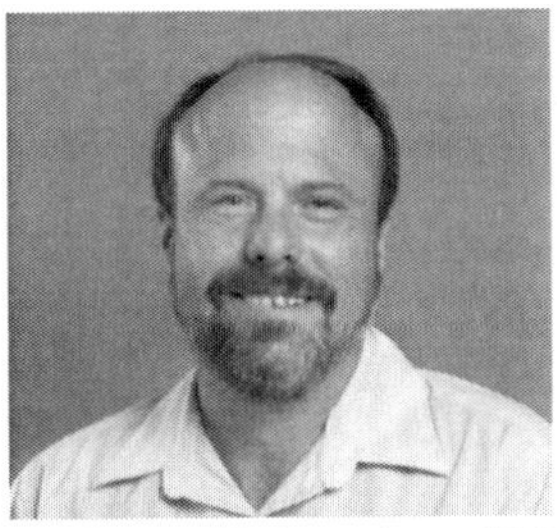

Department of Psychology, University of Missouri, Columbia, USA
SheldonK@missouri.edu

Ken Sheldon is a Professor of Social-Personality Psychology at the University of Missouri-Columbia. His primary research interests concern goals, motivation, creativity, and psychological well-being. He is also active in the "positive psychology" movement, having received a Templeton Prize in 2002 for his contributions to this emerging field. He has written six books, and more than 150 peer-reviewed articles. He pursues backpacking, photography, and tennis in his spare time.

Chapter 1

Mihaly Csikszentmihalyi

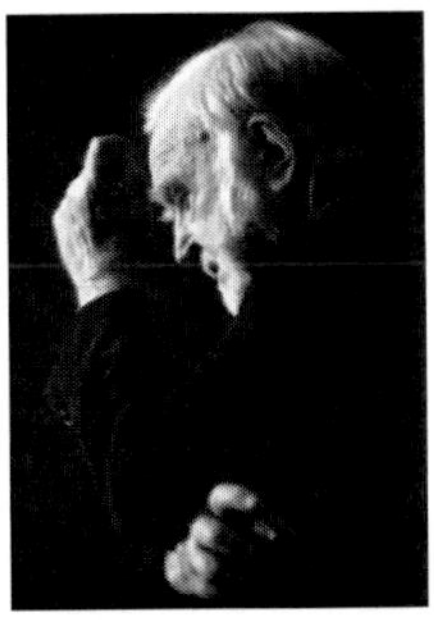

School of Behavioral and Organizational Sciences,
Claremont Graduate University, USA
miska@cgu.edu

Mihaly Csikszentmihalyi was born in Fiume, Italy (now Rijeka, Croatia), to Hungarian parents. He left Italy in 1956 to study in the United States. He received a PhD in Human Development from the University of Chicago in 1965, and started teaching at a nearby college. During this time, he developed the basic model of the flow experience.

In 1970 Mihaly was called back to the University of Chicago, where he became Chair of the Department of Psychology.

In 1999 he accepted an offer to teach at the Claremont Graduate University in California, where he started the first doctoral program in Positive Psychology.

Chapter 2

Martin I. Jones

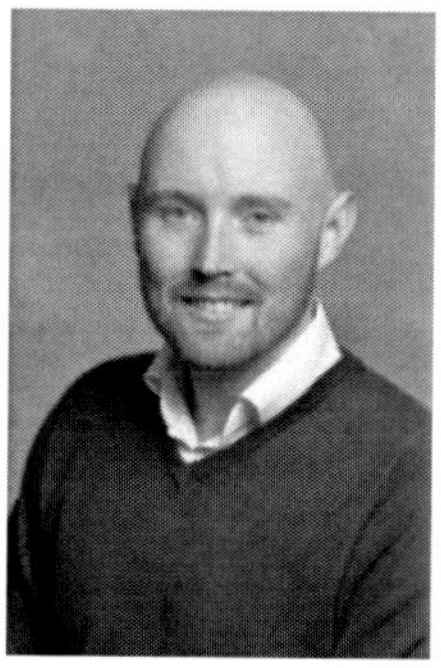

School of Sport & Exercise, University of Gloucestershire, UK
mjones2@glos.ac.uk

Martin is a senior lecturer in sport and exercise psychology at the University of Gloucestershire. Martin gained an MSc and PhD in sport psychology from Loughborough University and completed a Post-doctoral research fellowship in sport psychology at the University of Alberta Canada. Martin has published peer reviewed journal articles and book chapters on various topics in sport psychology including positive youth development, mental toughness, and sports coaching. Martin teaches sport and exercise psychology to undergraduate and postgraduate students and has received several student led teaching awards and a University of Gloucestershire teaching fellowship.

Since returning to the UK in 2010, Martin has become a British Association of Sport and Exercise Sciences Accredited Sport and Exercise Scientist, a Chartered Psychologist and an Associate Fellow of the British Psychological Society, a Science Council Chartered Scientist, a Fellow of the Higher Education Academy, and a Health and Care Professions Council registered sport and exercise psychologist.

John K. Parker

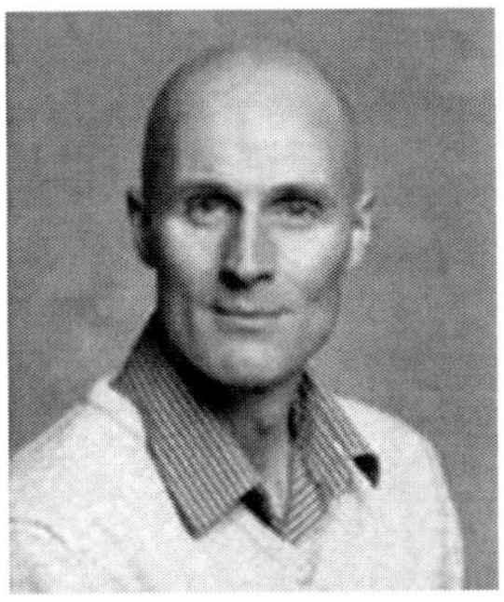

School of Sport & Exercise, University of Gloucestershire, UK

John is the course leader for the BSc sport and exercise sciences degree program at the University of Gloucestershire and a senior lecturer in sport and exercise psychology. John gained an MSc from Oxford Brookes University in cognitive neuropsychology and a PhD from the University of Gloucestershire in psychology. John has published research in imagery, youth sport, mental toughness, sports coaching, and exercise and cognition. John is a Chartered Psychologist and an Associate Fellow of the British Psychological Society, a Science Council Chartered Scientist, a Fellow of the Higher Education Academy, and a Health and Care Professions Council registered sport and exercise psychologist. John has coaching qualifications with the Professional Golfers Association and is an AA Class registered and a Fellow of the Professional Golfers Association.

Chapter 3

Terry Orlick

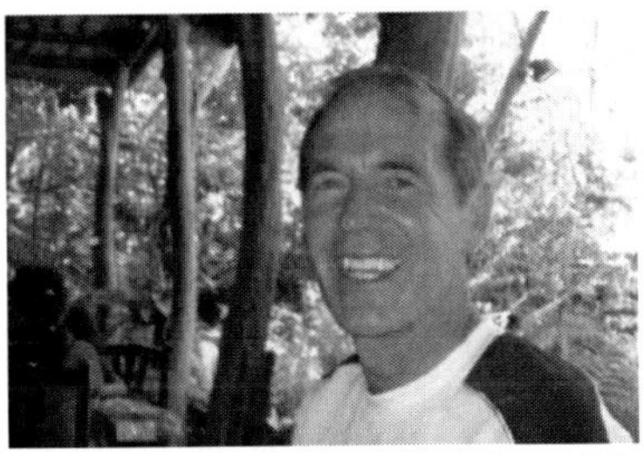

School of Human Kinetics, University of Ottawa, Canada
excel@zoneofexcellence.com

Dr Terry Orlick has been teaching university courses, supervising undergraduate and graduate students, conducting applied research and consulting with people of all ages to enhance their positive living skills, improve their positive focusing skills for sport and performance excellence and excel at quality living, at the University of Ottawa over the past 35 years. He has written over 20 books on Performance Excellence and Personal Excellence. His dream goal is help everyone on our planet (present and future) be what they have the potential to be, live the lives they would love to live, and help others live the positive lives they are capable of living.

Chapter 4

Daniel Gould

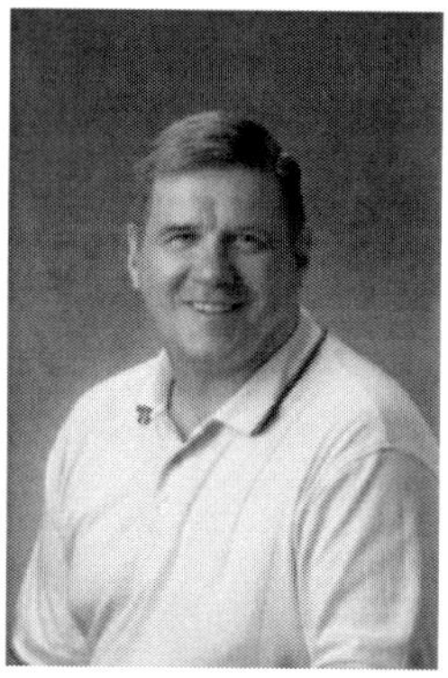

Institute for the Study of Youth Sports, Michigan State University, USA
drgould@msu.edu

Daniel Gould, PhD. Dan, is the Director of the Institute for the Study of Youth Sports and professor in the Department of Kinesiology at the Michigan State University. An active researcher, he has published more than 150 articles on sport psychology. Dan's current research focuses on the development of life skills, the psychology of coaching and parents in sport. He is best known for conducting applied research and for his efforts in coaching education. Dan is also actively involved in sport psychology consulting.

Scott Westfall

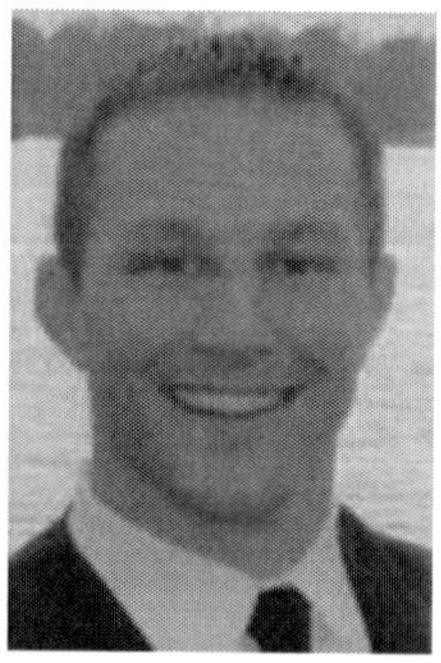

Institute for the Study of Youth Sports, Michigan State University, USA

Scott Westfall, M. Ed. After graduating from Colorado State University, Scott spent eight years as a teacher, coach, and athletic director at Boltz Middle School in Fort Collins, CO. Scott's main area of research focus is teaching life skills through sport. His hobbies include traveling, camping, skiing, rafting, boating, and spending time with his wife, Kelli.

Chapter 5

Tanya Forneris

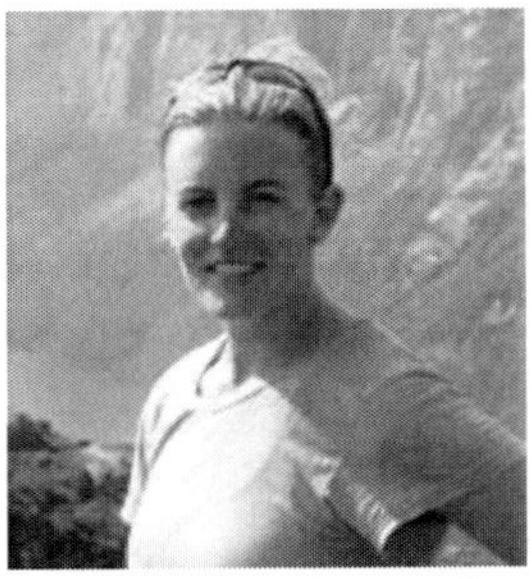

School of Human Kinetics, University of Ottawa, Canada
tforneri@uottawa.ca

Tanya Forneris, PhD, is an Associate Professor in the School of Human Kinetics at the University of Ottawa. Tanya's area of expertise is positive youth development and her research focuses on developing, implementing and evaluating community-based programming for youth. Tanya has worked extensively with various community organizations to help enhance the development of youth in Canada and abroad.

Tanya Halsall

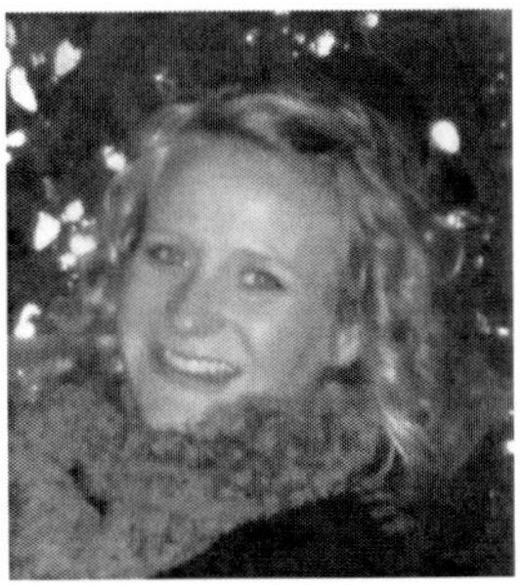

School of Human Kinetic, University of Ottawa, Canada

Tanya Halsall, MA, is a doctoral student in the School of Human Kinetics at the University of Ottawa. Tanya's primary research areas are in health promotion, program evaluation and community research with First Nations, Métis and Inuit youth. Her specific interests include the qualitative and quantitative study of interventions designed to improve well-being and psychological functioning.

Corliss Bean

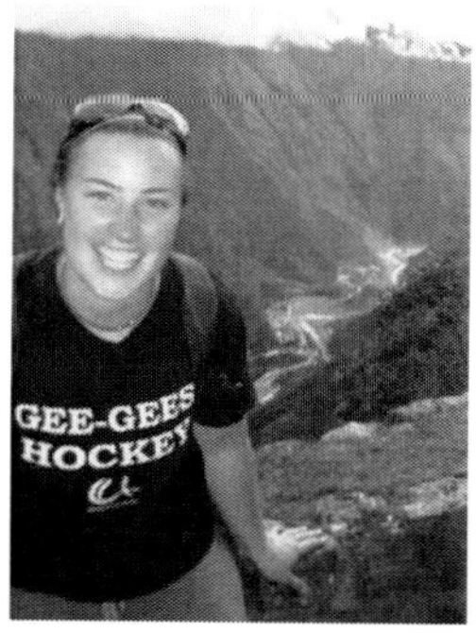

School of Human Kinetics, University of Ottawa, Canada

Corliss Bean, MA, is a doctoral student in the School of Human Kinetics at the University of Ottawa. Her research focuses on examining the impact of youth sport and physical activity programs on positive youth development, particularly with marginalized youth. Corliss is also the Research Coordinator for the Indigenous Health Research Group at the University of Ottawa.

Steven Danish

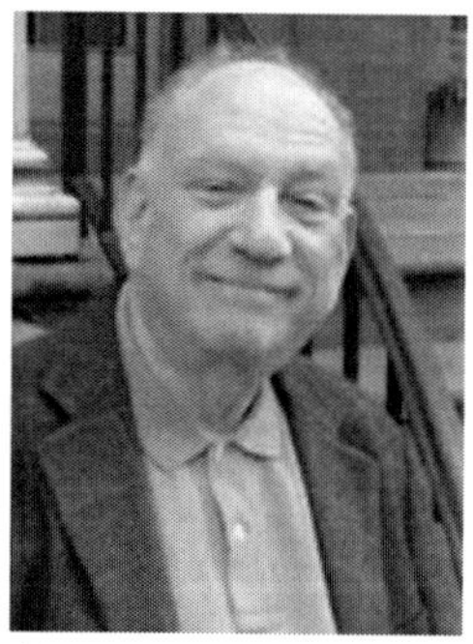

Department of Psychology. Virgnia Commonwealth University. USA.

Steven Danish, PhD, ABPP is the Director of the Life Skills Center and Professor of Psychology, at Virginia Commonwealth University. Steve has written over 120 articles and chapters in the areas of counseling, community and life span developmental psychology, sport psychology and military psychology. He was awarded the Lifetime Achievement award for "Prevention" by the Society for Counseling and received the distinguished Alumni Award from Michigan State University. Steve has also developed a number of award winning life skills programs for youth and adults.

Chapter 6

James E. Maddux

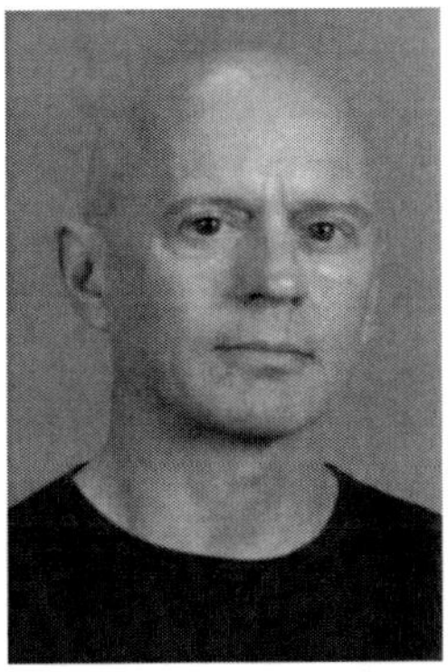

Department of Psychology. George Mason University. USA.
jmaddux@gmu.edu

James. E. Maddux is University Professor Emeritus of Psychology at George Mason University. He received his PhD in clinical psychology (with a minor in social psychology) from the University of Alabama in 1981. His major interest is the integration of theory and research from clinical, social, and health psychology. His research has been concerned primarily with understanding the influence of beliefs about personal effectiveness and control on psychological adjustment and health-related behavior. He is the former Editor of the *Journal of Social and Clinical Psychology* and former director of the clinical psychology doctoral program at George Mason University. He is the co-editor (with Barbara Winstead) of *Psychopathology: Foundations for a Contemporary Understanding* and (with June Tangney) *Social Psychological Foundations of Clinical Psychology*. Dr. Maddux is a Fellow of the American Psychological Association's Divisions of General, Clinical, and Health Psychology and a Fellow of the Association for Psychological Science. He also is a member of the Association of State and Provincial Psychology Board's Examination Committee, which is responsible for the Examination for the Practice of Professional Psychology used throughout the U.S. and Canada. In 2003 and 2004 he was a Guest Professor in the Department of Health Psychology at the Free University in Berlin.

Kimberley Dawson

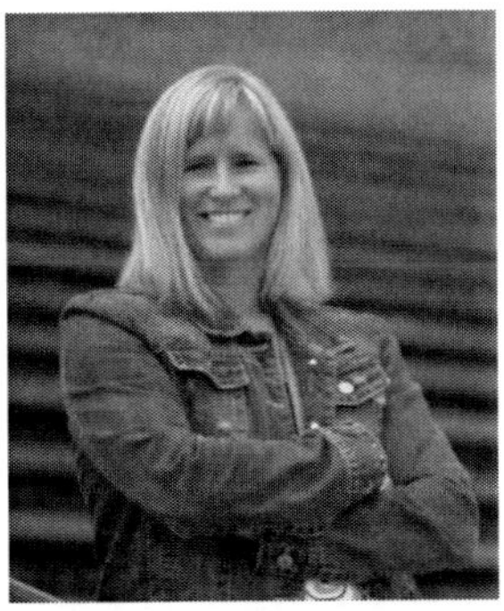

Department of Kinesiology and Physical Education,
Wilfrid Laurier University, Waterloo, Canada

Kim Dawson is a professor in Sport and Exercise Psychology in the Department of Kinesiology and Physical Education at Wilfrid Laurier University, Waterloo, Ontario, Canada. Her research interests involve understanding the social psychological influences that lead to behavior change in both the sport and exercise environments. Her main motivation is to increase the emotional well-being of both recreational and elite athletes and to help all individuals reach their full potential through physical activity and competition. Kim is also a member of the Canadian Sport Psychology Association and a recognized mental skills service provider by the Canadian Sport Institute. She is currently a performance psychology consultant for a number of sport organizations including Triathlon Canada and the Speed River Track & Field club where she helps athletes find the mental strength needed to maximize their physical capabilities.

Chapter 7

Kimberley L. Gammage

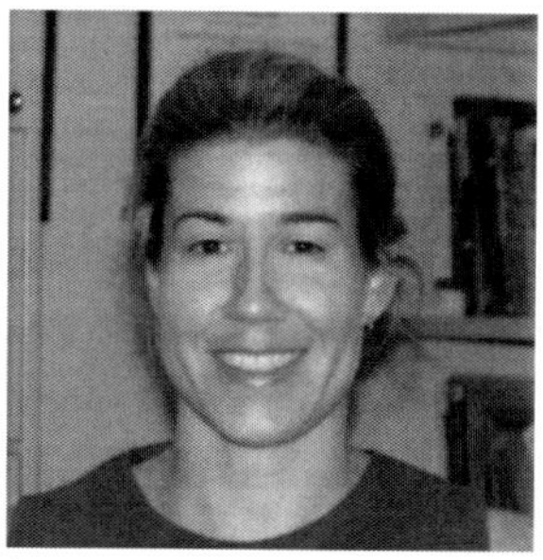

Department of Kinesiology, Brock University, St. Catharines, ON, Canada.
kgammage@brocku.ca

Kimberley Gammage is an Associate Professor at Brock University (Canada). Her research focuses on social-cognitive influences in exercise settings, including self-presentational concerns, body image and self-efficacy. As a group fitness instructor, she is particularly interested in how the exercise environment can be structured to maximize positive psychological outcomes and adherence. Her work also examines psychological influences on exercise in older adults, and she is director of a senior's exercise and balance program at Brock University.

Larkin Lamarche

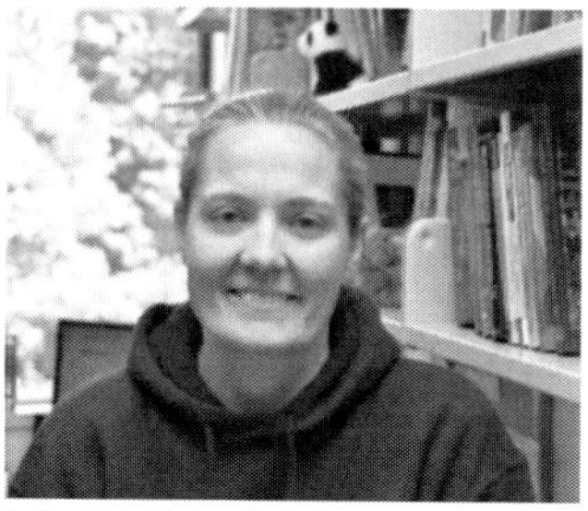

Department of Kinesiology, Brock University, St. Catharines, ON, Canada.

Larkin Lamarche is a post-doctoral fellow at Brock University (Canada). Her research is in the area of health and exercise psychology. She is particularly interested in body image and self-presentational concerns. Using a multidisciplinary approach to understanding body-related concerns, she is specifically interested in the psychobiology of body image experiences. She also investigates how psychological factors impact physical outcomes in balance and strength testing environments.

Chapter 8

Ali A. Weinstein

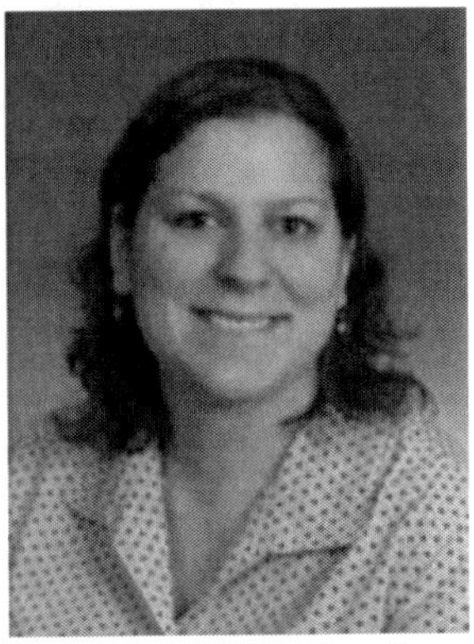

Center for the Study of Chronic Illness and Disability,
College of Health and Human Services, George Mason University, USA.
aweinst2@gmu.edu

Dr. Weinstein is an Associate Professor in the Department of Global and Community Health as well as the Deputy Director of the Center for the Study of Chronic Illness and Disability at George Mason University in Fairfax, VA. She holds a PhD in Medical Psychology and a Master's degree in Kinesiology (Sport/Exercise Psychology). Dr. Weinstein's research has focused on important contributors to health and recovery from illness and trauma: depression, stress, and physical activity/exercise.

Susan E. Lydick

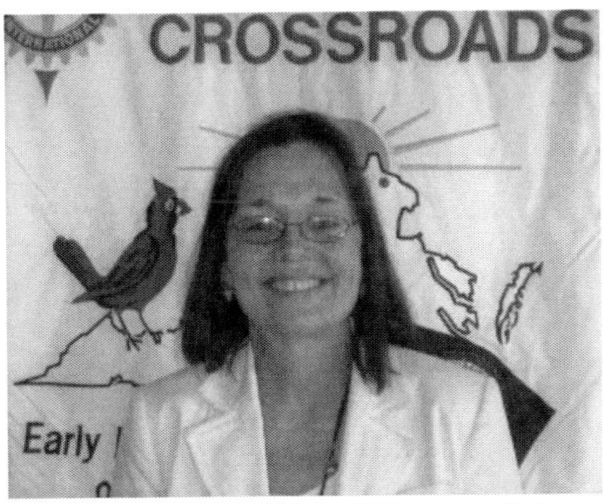

Department of Rehabilitation Science,
College of Health and Human Services,George Mason University, USA.

Ms. Lydick is a 3rd year doctoral student in the Department of the Rehabilitation Science at George Mason University. She earned her Master's degree in Psychology (Lifespan Development) at George Mason University and completed doctoral level coursework in Applied Developmental Psychology. Her research interests center around decreasing the impact of chronic stress, particularly traumatic stress, on long-term psychological and physical well-being.

Sukanya Biswabharati

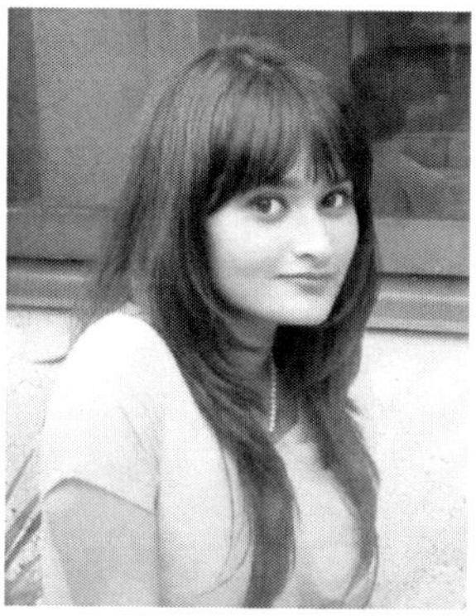

Department of Psychology and Biology, Faculty of Science, McMaster University, Canada.

Ms. Biswabharati is a recent graduate from McMaster University with a Bachelor of Science with Honours from the Department of Psychology and Biology. Her thesis investigated the audiovisual integration of biological motion in individuals with schizophrenia. She is currently pursuing her interests in various avenues of neuropsychology while preparing for medical school.

INDEX

#

A

B

C

D

G

H

I

J

K

L

M

N

O

P

Q

R

S

W

Y